YOUR AGING BODY CAN TALK

YOUR AGING BODY CAN TALK

Using Simple Muscle Testing to Learn What Your Body Knows and Needs **After 50**

Susan L. Levy, D.C.

Kalindi Press
Chino Valley, Arizona

© 2017, Peaceful Valley Retreat

All rights reserved. No part of this book may be reproduced in any manner without written permission from the publisher, except in the case of quotes used in critical articles and reviews.

Cover Design: Adi Zuccarello, adizuccarello.com

Interior Design and Layout: Becky Fulker, Kubera Book Design, Prescott, Arizona

Library of Congress Cataloging-in-Publication Data

Names: Levy, Susan, 1952- author.
Title: Your aging body can talk : using simple muscle testing to learn what your body knows and needs after 50 / Susan L. Levy, D.C.
Description: Chino Valley, Arizona : Kalindi Press, 2017. | Includes index.
Identifiers: LCCN 2016052586 | ISBN 9781935826453 (trade pbk.)
Subjects: LCSH: Applied kinesiology--Popular works. | Muscle strength--Testing. | Muscles--Aging.
Classification: LCC RZ251.A65 L47 2017 | DDC 613.7/1--dc23
LC record available at https://lccn.loc.gov/2016052586

Kalindi Press
P.O. Box 4410
Chino Valley, AZ 86323
800-381-2700
http://www.kalindipress.com

Disclaimer: Any information in this book is not intended to be a replacement for medical advice. Any person with a condition requiring medical attention should consult a qualified health professional.

This book was printed in the U.S.A. on recycled, acid-free paper using soy ink.

Dedication

This book is dedicated to my parents,
Allorah Jo and Sam.
You both gave me life, taught me to problem-solve
and to value learning.
Thank you.

Acknowledgements

Along the path of writing this book, many (too many to name) individuals have offered support to me and to this project.

A very special thank-you is in order for my niece, Chelsea. She spent countless hours at the keyboard, as well as, helping to polish and refine the text. Another thank you for keeping the most current version of the countless edits at the top of my inbox. Thank you for your efforts in research and documentation.

Thank you to Stacy Kitzman for producing the illustrations. I admire your artistic abilities.

I want to thank my editor, Regina Sara Ryan, for her help, support and guidance. I see you as my guiding light in this undertaking.

To Dasya Zucarello, publisher of Kalindi Press, thank you for your continued support and your efforts to bring this information to more and more readers.

I want to thank the many elders who have been my patients over a period spanning four decades. Thank you for sharing the essence of your being. Thank you all for sharing your wisdom and your rich life experiences. I have journeyed from young adulthood to embarking upon the path to elderhood along with some of you.

Coincident with the writing of this book, I have come to know dozens of wonderful people, some who live and others who work at an independent living community. This community has a friendly and genuinely caring culture, and truly strives to function as a community of wise elders. I feel privileged to have acquainted several wonderful people in this community, including two centenarians, Tudy and Al.

Thank you to my friends, for your support, and for listening to various passages needing revision.

Thank you to my entire family for your love and support, and for encouraging me to continue writing. I appreciate and love you all.

A special thank-you to my mother, Allorah Jo; you have shown us that deciding to downsize, to engage in a new community, and to readjust one's lifestyle is achievable.

May we together continue to learn how our aging bodies talk to us.

Contents

Introduction   xi
Chapter 1: Philosophy and Culture of Eldering   1
Chapter 2: Build Your Niche, Define Your Path   12
Chapter 3: Coming to Terms   19
Chapter 4: Move it and Preserve it   33
Chapter 5: Eat What You Are Made Of…   52
Chapter 6: …and Trash the Rest: Detoxing for Longevity   105
Chapter 7: Inflammation: The Anti-Youthing Agent   137
Chapter 8: Brain Longevity   157
Chapter 9: Youthing: Create Your Health and Longevity   176
Appendix: Muscle Testing Procedure   193
Index   195
Contact Information

Introduction

As our lives move through cycles of glorious sunrises and sunsets, we become older. I have written this book, *Your Aging Body Can Talk*, to bring a totally new concept, a life-changing approach to you. It is important for each individual to reflect upon the aging process and realize that their philosophy and beliefs about aging deeply affect the progression and outcome of that inevitable process. Today you can begin learning to incorporate proactive **youthing** thoughts and actions into your refreshing new lifestyle.

Youthing is a new word that I have coined to describe a proactive process of adding rich days and years to your life in the most youthful fashion possible. Believe that your body, and your entire being, flows from one rewarding life experience to the next with the least amount of wear and tear.

One path to accomplish this is to respectfully listen to your body and efficiently provide for its needs. In its infinite wisdom, your body consistently sends messages to you concerning its needs, its state of being, and which lifestyle factors either hamper or augment its function and its inherent quest for youthing.

Why Should You Read This Book?
This book is intended for everyone; after all each of us will hopefully walk the path of health well into our elder years. Whether you are already in your elder years, or are assisting your parents, grandparents, or elder loved ones along their journey, this book will delineate the path for aging in the most healthful and rewarding way possible.

You (and every person) should have easy access to such basic information as how your body functions, what your body needs, and how your body communicates its needs, likes, and dislikes. Both modern culture and modern medical practice have been hiding this valuable data from the public. It is time to pull back the curtain and reveal the truth to all.

In my natural healthcare wisdom and experience that has been building since the mid-1970s, the very best tool for understanding how you can help your body to optimize function and to minimize dysfunction is to become well acquainted with and very conversant with your own body. Clinical Kinesiology is my preferred method of communication to facilitate these ends.

Most people have never had such radical (nor such practical) advice from their doctor. It is time to proactively take control of your life, your health, and your future.

Using the vehicle of Clinical Kinesiology you can ferret out the truth about puzzling and confounding quandaries. Should I eat whole wheat bread? Should I eat a gluten-free diet? Is it in my best interests to eat fast food six times per week? Does my body respond with inflammation to foods and beverages I commonly consume? Is my immune system strong and balanced? Are five hours of sleep at night enough for me? Should I "rev" myself up with 3 cups of coffee in the morning and depend on sleeping pills at night? Am I a victim of my own self-limiting beliefs? Am I benefitting from my personal and social relationships? Are my current life goals appropriate for me? Am I accelerating the aging process in my body by adhering to misguided cultural expectations?

While your conscious mind may have logical and prudent answers to some of these questions, you and your body will get along best and be healthiest if you actually include your body and your entire being in the question and answer process. If you agree with this premise, you are a perfect candidate to begin learning basic Clinical Kinesiology testing techniques that you will find within this book.

What Will I Learn From Reading This Book?

The first chapter of this book (*Philosophy and Culture of Eldering*) will discuss various cultures and their philosophies about the aging process in order to reaffirm and strengthen your belief in your own wisdom.

As we move into Chapter 2 (*Build Your Niche, Define Your Path*), you will learn how to benefit from the idyllic principles just presented, and reconnect with the "real world" that you live in today. Perhaps the realities of your life today and the strength of your being will be the bricks, and the philosophical understandings will be the mortar of your new youthing lifestyle. This second chapter is meant to serve as the framework for defining your personal youthing practices and routines. Once you have established "your niche" and defined your path, we will explore new ways to consider improving your journey toward and through elderhood. Chapter 3 (*Coming To Terms*) will also empower you to come to terms with your own aging/youthing process and provide inspiration for how to proactively approach it.

Chapter 4 (*Move and Preserve It*) is all about physical mobility, exercise and honoring your body's limitations while still encouraging an active lifestyle in your older years. The next topics this book covers are best choices for your youthing diet and simple detoxification strategies in Chapters 5 (*Eat What You Are Made Of...*) and 6 (*...and Trash the Rest*). Chapter 7 (*Inflammation: The Anti-Youthing Agent*) discusses the common condition of inflammation in your older years and how to minimize it and live your life in the most youthful way possible.

Memory and brain health are discussed in Chapter 8 (*Brain Longevity*), and you will be provided with a wide array of tools and tips that guide you to maintain and encourage best cognitive brain performance. This book concludes (Chapter 9, *Youthing*) with a summary of the proactive measures that you can implement into your new "youthing" lifestyle as well as providing you a "roadmap" for creating your best personal universe in order to remain fulfilled and joyful as you age.

Throughout this book you will be reminded of your body's wisdom, your new tool to tap into that wisdom, and many ways to instill youthing measures into your daily life.

Why I Should Take Dr. Susan Levy's Advice?

As one of the world's most experienced and versatile natural healthcare providers, I have presented difficult subject matter in a simple manner that will allow you to live healthiest as you age and adopt your youthing lifestyle. I have studied countless natural healing methods, procedures, treatments and remedies. I have been a student of many of the most innovative and iconic natural healthcare practitioners from the 1980s to the present. Sadly, many of my mentors and teachers are no longer walking the earth, but I take my responsibility to preserve and record their legacy and bring this wealth of knowledge to the public very seriously.

I have completed formal training and certification or licensure in each of the following disciplines: nursing assistant, massage therapist, registered nurse, Cardiopulmonary Resuscitation (CPR), doctor of Chiropractic, diplomat in chiropractic orthopedics, and acupuncture. I have incessantly pursued the study of numerous other healing and diagnostic techniques including Clinical Kinesiology, numerous Chiropractic techniques, cranial manipulation, polarity therapy, nutrition, herbology, homeopathy, essential oils, various body-mind techniques, light therapy, sound and music therapy, visual imagery and various energy medicine techniques.

I began working in the healthcare arena in 1970 as a nursing assistant, in 1974 as a registered nurse. Soon I was intrigued with the natural approach to health and wellness and began studying herbology and massage therapy as I reentered college to take additional chemistry and science courses as a prerequisite for entering Chiropractic College.

As a private practitioner, I have involved my patients in problem solving for their various health issues since 1981. I have learned from each of them. I continuously undertake postgraduate studies and continuing education courses.

My gift to the public at large is my first book *Your Body Can Talk*. It is a handbook for understanding your body and how to communicate with it. My gift to those interested in learning how to be kind to yourself as you grow older is *Your Aging Body Can Talk*.

What Is Clinical Kinesiology?

It is an innovative technique to delve into understanding your body and its physiology. In this application, you are your own diagnostic instrument. The technique involves using your own healthy and intact muscles, usually an uninjured arm or leg. For our purposes, a strong muscle group (your straight and extended arm) is tested for inherent strength. If it is unhampered, it can be tested while various questions about your body's functions, or its compatibility with external objects or substances are evaluated. In essence, Clinical Kinesiology uses movement and function of your body to extract information from your internal database.

Clinical Kinesiology was developed by Dr. Alan Beardall in the late 1900s to monitor and test the energetic systems of the body based on muscle testing. The Clinical Kinesiology method concentrates on organ and physiological relationships as they correlate to certain muscle reflexes, as well as the link between mind, body, and spirit. Dr. Beardall also discovered the exciting relationship of handmodes (specific hand and finger positions) and their relationship to our physiology and or organ systems. When the hand or fingers are placed in certain positions or are touching certain areas of the body, the body will give a strong (positive) or a weak (negative) response with the indicator muscle (the opposite arm or leg that is being used for testing).

Clinical Kinesiology is a noninvasive modality that utilizes muscle testing, handmodes, and other means to diagnose and discover underlying imbalances within the body. Since Dr. Beardall's initial breakthrough, hundreds of handmodes have been discovered as "words" in this new language of the body. Clinical Kinesiology is an effective diagnostic tool that can be used to determine dis-ease, energy blockages, as well as to help establish the best means of treatment and healing.

Clinical Kinesiology is a simple and user-friendly tool to assist you in making your best lifestyle choices on a daily basis. The following excerpt from *Your Body Can Talk, 2nd Edition* is illustrative.

> *Dr. Alan Beardall's Clinical Kinesiology method relies on the extremely precise energy connection between mind and body. Your body has been pre-programmed to sustain life. Each cell, body part, organ and energy system is genetically encoded to work for continued survival of the organism. Your brain acts as*

a giant "switching" center to channel this energy into action to maintain body function, coordinate messages, store data and retrieve information. As connections are made, energy flows and intelligence is communicated. Your body "talks," thus the "tapping in" to this communication through muscle testing "works."

The brain processes information precisely like a binary (functioning on a system of "two") computer systematically turning "on" or "off" in relation to any given subject, or perception. Based on the Clinical Kinesiology test, we're looking for a "lock" or neurological reflex that's "on" or "off." This makes a muscle test that is strong (on) or weak (off) a simplistic, yet invaluable diagnostic tool.

*If I say to you, "**Do not think** about pink elephants," **you have to think** about pink elephants! I just turned "on" the pink elephant switch in your brain. It will stay on until your brain determines the next priority, or the next important thing that it needs to think about. Then, you'll drop the "pink elephants" and move on.*[1]

How Do I Begin?

The foundational step for beginning to use Clinical Kinesiology or muscle response testing is to maintain a perfectly neutral mind. This means to earnestly be in an open-minded state, avoiding preconceived ideas and preferences. Give yourself the responsibility of being a scientist looking for the true answer. Dr. Alan Beardall consistently instructed his students "search for the truth". You should also follow that instruction.

Make provisions for a healthful, quiet and unobtrusive environment for testing. Do your best to choose an area free from excessive noise, electronic equipment, noxious odors, temperature extremes and the like.

Be sure you are not dehydrated, by drinking a glass of water shortly before testing. This helps your brain and nervous system to function at best.

Be sure you have a sturdy and comfortable chair to sit in and all anticipated materials (such as food, beverages, supplements or herbs to be tested) close at hand.

Be sure to have available one or two items to test that are likely to be incompatible with your body in order to validate the presence or absence of a weak muscle response to a known toxin. Examples could be dish soap, powdered cleanser, or even a packet of sugar or artificial sweetener.

Practice testing yourself several times to gain comfort with the process. Essentially, each muscle test is a question and the muscle response is its answer.

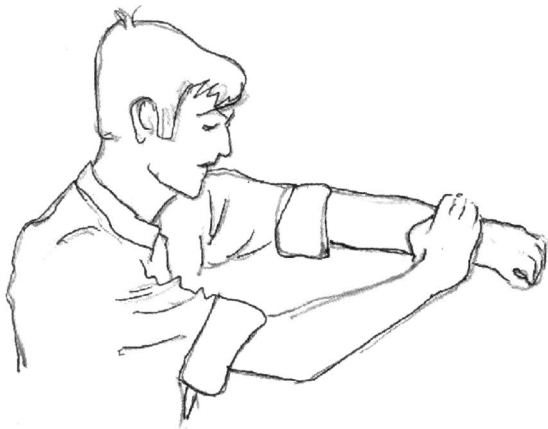

For a review and for quick reference, a summary of the muscle testing procedure follows.

Muscle Testing Procedure

Clinical Kinesiology muscle testing is a simple and effective tool that can aid in your ability to understand the language of your body. You may wish to seek out a professional Clinical Kinesiologist in order to perform detailed muscle testing, but for more generalized and basic questions you can perform self-testing by following simple steps.
- Sit in a comfortable and sturdy chair.

(continued)

- Remember to maintain a neutral state of mind.
- Perform an "indicator muscle test"* to determine your baseline strength by pushing on your dominant arm with your other hand. If you can easily resist moderate pressure, rest and then proceed.
- In order to test a food, supplement or similar item, you can place the item in your hand, lap or pocket and test for compatibility using the same format as the indicator muscle test.
  - If your body responds with a "strong" muscle test, you know that the food or supplement is compatible with your body.
  - If you find a "weak" muscle test in which your arm is easily pushed downward, you should avoid the food or other item.

* Indicator Muscle Test *

To perform an indicator muscle test, or test your arm's strength, hold one arm straightforward at shoulder height, parallel to the floor. Place the outstretched fingers on the other hand just slightly above the wrist of your testing arm. Keep the palm and fingers of the testing hand flat, just resting above the other wrist, not clutching it. Firmly hold the testing arm stationary as you then push down or toward the floor with the other (the pushing) hand. If you want to test yourself for compatibility with a food or supplement hold the item in your testing hand (the straight arm), or place it in your pocket. You should be able to discern between a weak and a strong muscle response. I strongly advise doing several practice tests to get the feel of the process.[2]

By following these instructions, you can gain insight into your own body's wisdom. You can also learn about what it truly needs.

LEARN MORE

To review more detailed methods of self testing and learn more about Clinical Kinesiology, refer to Chapter 1 in *Your Body Can Talk, 2nd Edition* by Susan L. Levy, D.C.

Books

Levy, Susan L., D.C. *Your Body Can Talk, Second Edition*. Chino Valley, Ariz: Kalindi Press, 2014.

Endnotes, Introduction

1. Levy, Susan L., D.C. *Your Body Can Talk, Second Edition*. Chino Valley, Ariz: Kalindi Press, 2014, 5-6.
2. Ibid., 17.

CHAPTER 1

Philosophy and Culture of Eldering

Benita wakes before her rooster crows each day. She gives thanks for her life and her blessings. She stretches, quickly changes from her nightgown to a vibrantly colored skirt and blouse, and begins her morning chores. She tidies up the two-room home that she shares with Guillermo, her husband of eighty years. Yes, that's right, eighty years of marriage. Benita is 105 and Guillermo is 106. They are both semisupercentenarians (persons between 105 and 109 years old).

When Guillermo rises, his first chores are feeding his chickens and collecting their freshly laid eggs, checking the prevailing wind direction, and tending the garden. Just after sunrise, he brings the eggs and the daily harvest of vegetables into their roughly planked, wooden home.

By 6:00 A.M., Benita is already busy grinding corn for their tortillas and boiling beans and squash. Just like her mother, grandmother, and great grandmother had done, Benita makes her tortillas from corn that has been prepared by soaking in water with wood ash and lime to facilitate grinding. This process improves the nutrient value of the corn by adding minerals, especially calcium. Adding the enriched water helps facilitate protein digestion.[1]

For generations, Benita's and Guillermo's families have lived in Hojancha, a small village on the Península de Nicoya, on the Pacific coast of Costa Rica. Benita's ancestors were the Chortega Indians indigenous to Nicoya.[2] Their simple, yet purposeful way of life, and their basic and nutritious diet continues to enrich the Chortega Indian descendants, today's Nicoyan people. These sturdy, industrious folks are famous for their longevity.[3]

Shortly after a simple breakfast of homemade tortillas, beans and rice, Guillermo and Benita go to work in the garden that they describe as their "personal Eden." It is filled with a dozen lush fruit trees of many varieties, including the exotic fruit *marañón,* which is extremely high in vitamin C, and *anona,* a fruit known to have cancer-preventing properties. Benita and Guillermo also have rows of fresh vegetables, edged by their corn and bean fields. They pull weeds by hand from their exquisite garden, seemingly oblivious to the use of toxic pesticides or chemical-laden weed killers.

Each Sunday, Benita prepares an elaborate meal of foods collected from her garden and orchard for her children, grandchildren and great grandchildren who remain in the small Hojancha village. Guillermo looks lovingly at his wife, and often expresses his affection with a brief kiss and hug as he passes through their kitchen where she and the other women prepare the meal.

Modern-day researchers have found that having a secure sense of purpose is a significant contributor to longevity and health. Together, Benita and Guillermo carry out numerous purposeful and necessary tasks each day. They depend on each other to carry out their designated tasks and rely on one another's love, support and companionship. We can all learn about the vital importance of purposeful living from their example.

Elders Respected in Traditional Cultures Around the World
Geronta is a term of endearment applied to the monks at the ancient monastery called Tharri on the island of Rhodes in Greece.[4] This term is traditionally used to address the monks in a reverent, respectful fashion. *Gerondassa* translates to mean "old man." But this usage has no negative connotation of weakness or inability. Quite conversely, referring to a monk as an "old man" is considered complementary and implies that the speaker acknowledges the monk's wisdom, experience, and closeness to God. *Gerontissa,* the feminine form of this word, is reserved for elder nuns who spiritually guide others with their wise knowledge.

In the Greek tradition, and particularly in the Greek Orthodox religious domain, respect for the elders is second nature.

Many Asian cultures have rich traditions of respect and deference to elders. In the Korean tradition, the entire extended family prepares a grand celebration for family elders on their sixtieth and seventieth birthdays. *Hwan-gap* is the name of the sixtieth birthday celebration, and is a joyous event for the elders, their children, and their grandchildren. The celebration marks a life passage, the passage into older age. Upon achieving their seventieth birthday, the *kohCui*, or "old and rare" festivity is celebrated.

Similarly, traditional Chinese families highly value, respect, and express filial piety for their elders. In fact, honoring one's elders, as well as one's ancestors, is one of the highest virtues in this culture. Going against the wishes of the elders, disappointing one's elders, or showing disrespect for one's elders disgraces both the innocent elder and the younger offender with dishonor.

In rural and traditional China, placing a parent or grandparent into a retirement home or nursing home would be considered disrespectful and dishonorable. Families feel an obligation to lovingly care for their elders and welcome them to live with the extended family, regardless of inherent challenges.

The Okinawan traditions concerning their older generations and deceased ancestors are well defined and entrenched in the culture. The traditional religion of Okinawa, Ryukyuan, calls for celebration and commemoration of the lives of deceased ancestors for many years after their passing. Eventually, their original religious tradition was combined with Confucianism, Buddhism and the Shinto faith. The veneration of Okinawan ancestors has roots in each of the religious traditions that have come to their island. Deep regard and respect for living elders is an integral part of the Okinawan culture that continues into modern times.

For centuries in India, the eldest generation has been considered the head of the family and the multi-generational household. Younger generations would consult their elders for advice on all-important issues. While many of these virtues are rapidly changing as the subcontinent embraces the technology and culture of the West, it is still common for grandparents and great-grandparents to be involved in the nurturing and raising of the grandchildren while the parents work. Grandparents and great-grandparents are generally held in high regard, and are thought to hold the answers to all life's dilemmas.

On the North American continent, over 500 Native American nations are known. Each of these particular nations, often referred to as "tribes," has developed their own tradition and customs regarding human aging and care and respect for elders. The knowledge, experience, and wisdom of the elders have guided and molded daily life for each of these tribes for centuries. Though vastly different in many other respects, one consistent custom of all Native American tribes is the reliance upon elders to pass down tribal lore, tradition, and customs through the art of storytelling. Younger generations are urged to rely on their elders to teach them about their cultural identity though oral tradition in order to preserve tribal heritage and customs.

Within the Jewish culture, the Hebrew word for "old" is *zakein*, which translates as "wise." Religious custom and cultural protocol command that Jewish people respect all elders because of their rich life experience, tribulations, and successful problem-solving abilities that far outreach the experiences of younger generations. The idea that each additional year of life yields greater wisdom is a well-accepted fact in Jewish culture. Another example of heartfelt respect being shown to elders within this tradition is found with the recitation of the Kaddish prayer, which is a powerful adoration of the "Eternal One," as well as a commemoration of deceased ancestors and loved ones. The Kaddish prayer links the deceased to their Creator and reminds the living to honor their ancestors for the good acts and deeds of their departed loved ones. It is recited by the Rabbi and the congregation each Sabbath, and at special holidays throughout the year. Mourners who have lost a loved one during the week prior to a particular Sabbath show their respect by rising during the recitation of the Kaddish prayer. Those recently departed are honored as their names are read aloud during the sacred prayer. The *yahrzeit* marks each yearly anniversary of the loved one's passing. In addition to reciting the Kaddish prayer at the loved one's *yahrzeit*, mourners typically observe several strictly-adhered-to traditions such as covering mirrors in the home during the mourning period, frequently visiting the grave, and placing a small stone on the headstone as an eternal maker of the visit. These traditions and protocols exemplify the love and respect for one's ancestors (and other relatives and friends).

After a brief look at this sampling of various cultures whose traditions are steeped in honoring and respecting elders and their wisdom, it becomes obvious that the more recent emphasis of preferentially valuing youth and discounting elders and their rich experience is a fairly new twist in human cultural expression. This seems to have become more pronounced after the conclusion of World War II.

The modern era was ushered in by significant changes in cultural norms, behaviors and mores. By the early 1950s, televisions were present in more and more homes. Addictive behaviors, such as cigarette and cigar smoking and excessive alcohol use were common and could be viewed on the television screen on a daily basis.

The gruesome violence and carnage of the Vietnam War was seen in both still photographs and video format in all media forms. Movies and television shows have progressively portrayed graphic violence and disregard for human life from the late 1940s to the present.

Families became more fragmented and more mobile, often placing geographical rifts between grandparents and grandchildren, as well as adult siblings, at a rate accelerated more than ever before in history.

Stake Your Claim

What can we learn from a brief study of these ancient cultures? How can we apply even a few kernels of useful data into or own "becoming elder" process? Of course we could elect to study further and unearth more information; however, with the examples presented here it is obvious that the historical viewpoint of many diverse human cultures is that elders have been celebrated, loved, embraced, learned from, acknowledged, respected, and cared for as they progress through the later and even the final stages of their lives. Typically, this experience has been sweetened and peppered with wisdom, tools for refining judgment, and examination of an array of philosophical viewpoints, by all family or village members who care to participate. With this premise established, it behooves all who are treading (or even just stepping on to) the path to elderhood to stake our claims to meaningful elderhood, and focus or refocus on our life's purpose. This book will help you in staking that claim! And more, it will provide you with tools, and ways to evaluate and make better life choices.

Declare Your Inherent Self-Worth

Much in the same way certain monetary instruments—certificates of deposit and treasury bills—achieve their greatest value at maturity, so do your accrued set of life experiences and your wisdom enrich and mature. Now is a perfect time to reflect upon your own ethnic, religious, spiritual and cultural traditions, and give them new life. You may also examine your own principles and values, your attributes and your accomplishments. Have you fully acknowledged yourself as a wise elder? Could others benefit from sharing in your wisdom? How can you best share these treasures?

One way to honor your elderhood is by writing or recording your life's story. This exercise may be rewarding for you and inspiring to others. You may find a very personal way to commemorate your life's journey.

Now is also a perfect time to reminisce about treasured family traditions and the stories of your ancestors. I know a woman who enlarged and framed several of her mother's handwritten recipe cards and gave them to various family members to hang in their kitchens. Perhaps you can polish or give new life to your own memories, family stories and heirlooms. You may choose to have a "Sharing Memories" event with your friends and contemporaries, or with interested members of your family. You could have a tea party using your great aunt's newly polished silver tea service, make cookies or muffins using your mother's recipe and prepare a memory book of photos and stories of these matriarchs. If it is too challenging to create such an event, you can imagine and relish the memories and warm feelings you would like to relive.

Another idea is to spend a day or two at or near the area where your family vacationed, camped, fished or hiked in your childhood years. You could remember and relive exhilarating times that are still meaningful to you because of the ancestral connection and the positive feelings evoked by the surroundings.

The next step may be to consider how to open constructive two-way communications between the generations of your family and to find meaningful ways to engage younger family members in their family and cultural treasures and traditions.

We can each reflect upon how the elders that have preceded us have likely been a rich resource to guide us in learning life's lessons. We can all hope to be seen in that light by younger members of our family. We may not know what type of positive impact we have had on our descendents during our lifetime; nonetheless, it is a valuable exercise to make our best effort at being a desirable role model and conduit for our family and cultural legacies. As we explore and reaffirm our creative contributions to life we can enhance our health, wellness and longevity while providing emotional and cultural nurturance to ourselves and others.

Now is also a wonderful time to consider how we connect with our inner selves. Often we rush through life so quickly and in such a state of detachment that our very being is actually energetically fragmented rather than being fully connected and engaged.

Many of us living in today's world struggle to define our life's path, our self worth, or even to understand our cultural roots. Let's look at an ancient tool to give us direction and to reaffirm our life's purpose.

Define Your Life's Purpose and Live It

The Okinawans developed a seemingly simple and powerful method for staying fully aware, connected and engaged in their own lives. This beneficial method of staying focused and positively tuned-in is termed *ikigai*, pronounced eek-ee-guy. This ancient word means "the reason for which you get up in the morning," or alternatively, your personal sense of purpose. Within the traditional Okinawan culture, the norm was and is to have a clearly defined *ikigai*, but a person may redefine their *ikigai* whenever and as often as they choose.

Typically, Okinawans awake to the call of their *ikigai* and a resolute sense of their life's purpose even during their nineties and beyond. Often one's *ikigai* is attached strongly to their family, work or profession, or their hobbies or interests. Researchers conclusively found direct relationships between a person pursuing their *ikigai* and:
1. Measurably stronger immune-system markers
2. Diminished stress hormone levels
3. A more easygoing attitude and a greater ability to accommodate to unforeseen challenges and mishaps
4. Measurable longevity increases

In his book, *The Blue Zones: 9 Lessons for Living Longer from the People Who've Lived the Longest*, Dan Buettner writes: "Older Okinawans can readily articulate the reason they get up in the morning. Their purpose-embedded lives give them clear roles of responsibility and feelings of being needed well into their 100s."[5]

How to Define My Life's Purpose
Many people move through life from one activity to the next, from one priority to the next, and from one emergency to the next. If you have moved through life in this fashion, you likely have not taken the time to define your life's purpose. Now is the time to do this; it's never too late. You are the author of your life's purpose. You are the only person who can define it, decree it and live it. This important project essentially has no rules. You can take several days or weeks to formulate your first go at naming your life's purpose, and then perhaps even decide to change it the next day.

If this is a new process for you, realize that it will take extra thought and discernment. It is best to approach this endeavor in a calm and relaxed fashion.

You may not have answers for each of these points, but simply considering these components of your life will begin to bring you closer to defining your *ikigai*.

As you read and reread the lists, you may get clues to your life's purpose and you should highlight or place asterisks by the entries that

> **Searching for My *Ikigai***
> 1. Write a list of the things you most enjoy in life.
> 2. Write a list of your favorite accomplishments.
> 3. Write a list of how you most enjoy spending your time.
> 4. Write a list of your most treasured values.
> 5. Write a list of actions or activities you would miss most if unable to pursue them.
> 6. Write a list of the most important relationships in your life: family, friends, colleagues, mentors, etc. Consider writing briefly about what these relationships mean to you and how you want to contribute to them.
> 7. Write a list of salient points to potentially include in your autobiography (whether or not you ever write it)

most strike a chord with your inner self. You can then select several of these and write them individually on small slips of paper or 3x5 cards.

Please review the instructions for the Muscle Testing Procedure on pages xvii and xviii of the Introduction.

Drink a glass of water and be certain that your environment is comfortable and peaceful. Sit in a comfortable chair for doing your self-testing. Have your 3x5 cards easily accessible to you, but be sure to turn the cards facedown before you begin testing.

Sit in a comfortable and sturdy chair.

Remember to maintain a neutral state of mind.

Perform an Indicator Muscle Test (page xviii) to determine your base-line strength by pushing on your dominant arm with your other hand. If you can easily resist moderate pressure, rest and then proceed.

Take one 3x5 card and place it in your pocket or on your lap and then test this activity for compatibility in the same format as you used for the Indicator Muscle Test.

If your body responds with a "strong" muscle test, you know that the potential activity or endeavor is compatible with your life's purpose. It's a Keeper; place it in a pile to further reference in determining your *ikigai*.

If you find a "weak" muscle test, your arm is easily pushed downward; this factor is probably not currently a component or clue to your *ikigai*. Discard it, or put it aside. It will not be needed.

When complete with each of your cards, consider the components that produced a strong or positive muscle test. Each of these likely is quite important to your inner being, and may be a clue to the formulation of your *ikigai*. Reflect on these clues, and use them to jumpstart the articulation of your life's purpose.

When you feel that you are close to having defined your life's purpose, by all means write it down and date it. Read and review your written *ikigai* frequently and feel free to modify or change it as you please.

Listening to Your Body's Wisdom
The people in the previously described cultures relied on the wisdom of their own body . . . they had to, for survival! They listened to how their bodies desired to interact with their native environments. For example, the story of Benita and Guillermo illustrates how many traditional peoples are tuned-in to their bodies, daily customs, and environment enough to awaken just before sunrise to maximize the benefit of daylight, and to retire to bed at dark for optimal sleep and rejuvenation. Other groups throughout the ages have lived in harmony with the constant movement of day and night, seasonal changes, and seasons of life changes. Commonly, those with extended lifespan have been privileged to eat fresh, locally grown and/or raised foods, and these foods were certainly not tainted with GMOs, pesticides, preservatives, dyes, or other toxins, as they are today.

Many readers do not have the luxury of a pristine and simple lifestyle, but instead live in a technologically-advancing, industrial world where choices are so abundant that sometimes it may be hard to discern the healthiest options in lifestyle orientation or food choices, along with what healing methods are best suited to their ongoing strength, happiness and longevity. Clinical Kinesiology, on which this book is based, provides those of us who may not live such an intuitively guided lifestyle with an accurate and easy-to-use methodology that teaches us to understand our body's language and tune into its true, healthy desires.

Today, many of us have more accessible knowledge and resources available to allow us to make the best choices for ourselves and our decedents. Let us all make wise and informed choices. As we move forward in our journey to and through elderhood, we each face personal and unique challenges. The next chapter will help you build your own niche in our ever changing world.

LEARN MORE

Books

Beare, Sally. *50 Secrets of the World's Longest Living People, Expanded Ed Edition.* Boston: Da Capo Press, 2005.

Buettner, Dan. *The Blue Zones, Second Edition: 9 Lessons for Living Longer from the People Who've Lived the Longest.* Washington, D.C.: National Geographic Society, 2012.

Pevny, Ron. *Conscious Living, Conscious Aging: Embrace and Savor Your Next Chapter.* New York: Atria Paperback, 2014.

Robbins, John. *Healthy at 100: The Scientifically Proven Secrets of the World's Healthiest and Longest-Lived Peoples.* New York: Ballantine Books, 2007.

Tolle, Eckhard. *A New Earth 10th Anniversary Edition: Awakening to Your Life's Purpose.* Westminster, London: Penguin Random House, 2008.

Endnotes, Chapter 1

1. Buettner, Dan. *The Blue Zones, Second Edition: 9 Lessons for Living Longer from the People Who've Lived the Longest.* Washington, D.C.: National Geographic Society, 2012. 195.
2. Ibid., 192.
3. Ibid.
4. "7 Cultures That Celebrate Aging and Respect Elders." *The Huffington Post.* 2015. http://www.huffingtonpost.com/2014/02/25/what-other-cultures-can-teach_n_4834228.html
5. Buettner, 118.

CHAPTER 2

Build Your Niche, Define Your Path

Our virtual trip to visit rural Costa Rica, Okinawa, and ancient Japan to sample the cultural respect and reverence for elders of yore has been refreshing. Today, we must each carve out our individual "elder niche" within our own local area or culture, and in some cases, even within our own families. As we grow to cherish our life's wisdom, we step into the place and the role of "wise elder" with ourselves and for others.

Since for many folks this sense of *ikigai* has been neglected or forgotten, the first step in this growing-wisdom process is to review your life's purpose or *ikigai* and then revise and/or polish it if needed. This will help you to see how your life impacts your family, friends, various social, political and spiritual groups, and even the world. Now that instantaneous communication and news transmission is inherently woven into life's fabric, you can more easily understand the human connection from a global perspective.

Each of our actions and even our thoughts has the power to affect the world around us. As our individual pursuits augment the greater good of humanity, even while interacting with one or two people we define our own niche as a respected elder. For example, if you hold the door open for an elder with mobility challenges and greet them with a smile or pleasant "hello," all observers will learn from your example. Perhaps they will soon be opening doors and conversing with others whom they encounter, and maybe you will be the recipient of their kindness down the road.

Leaving Your Mark

You *can* move beyond simply defining your life's purpose. This chapter also aims to encourage you to "leave your mark" on the world and those around you by both nurturing and disciplining yourself towards the goal of achieving the greatest "you" that you can manifest. That expanded sense of self-appreciation, love and purpose will then touch everyone you come into contact with. It may or may not include a physical legacy to pass on, but your "mark" will be made nonetheless.

During this mark-building and manifesting process you may choose to read and study, in greater depth, topics that you are already familiar with. You may find this to be a perfect time in your life to undertake study of new topics and activities, simply for the joy of self-enrichment or as a means to serve others.

"Leaving your mark" could be in any realm of human endeavor. You may choose from disciplines such as writing poetry, studying and documenting your own ancestral genealogy, learning to can or dehydrate fruits and vegetables for future use, ballroom dancing, becoming a docent at your local art museum, learning a new language or volunteering at a charity service. You might determine to "leave your mark" by simply becoming a person of greater inner wisdom through prayer and contemplation. Leaving your mark does not require that the world take notice, simply that you experience a comfortable degree of self-fulfillment.

My mother, Allorah Jo, has spent years studying genealogy. She and one of her brothers searched out several ancestral family lines. They traced one line back to the year 1408 in Italy, and another one back to the year 1066 in Ireland. These explorations were rewarding and were a means for the brother and sister to connect to each other and with their shared ancestral past. They submitted their discoveries to the Family History Library, and the information is preserved at familysearch.org. Now our family heritage can easily be shared by living decedents and by generations to come.

Wisdom and Achievements Expressed after Fifty

Grandma Moses began her artistic career at the age of seventy-eight, Laura Ingalls Wilder wrote and published her popular *Little House* books in her sixties, and the world famous chef Julia Child didn't launch her popular television show until she was fifty.

Ernie Andrus, a World War II veteran, ran west to east across America. He began his journey on October 7, 2013 in San Diego. He concluded his cross-country run on August 20, 2016 at St. Simon's Island, Georgia, one day after his ninety-third birthday.

While these examples of famous people are often cited, I think we all know others in our families or communities who are still practicing art, music, service and active kindness well into their elder years. It's never too late to begin.

- "O Lord, keep me alive as long as I live."—Old Scottish Prayer
- "It is never too late to be what you might have been." —George Eliot
- "I began a midlife corporate career at age 53, started modeling at 63, and became a published author and speaker at 68." —Valerie Ramsey
- "If we don't change, we don't grow. If we don't grow, we aren't really living."—Gail Sheehy

---

Using Clinical Kinesiology to Find Your Potential

With so many possible life-enriching activities or enjoyable challenges to choose from, it is helpful to narrow the field by first writing a list of possible new endeavors that pique your interest. Next, spend a few days reviewing and editing your list, adding and deleting entries, and then circling or highlighting the most intriguing and achievable choices. Keep in mind any potentially limiting factors, such as mobility, energy requirements, climatic and financial considerations.

The next step will be to write each of the likely prospects on a 3x5 card and then proceed to use your new Clinical Kinesiology skills to further evaluate. You will be using Clinical Kinesiology as a tool to help you determine which of these engaging activities are most closely in tune with your inner self.

Muscle Testing for New Endeavors
Review the instructions for performing Clinical Kinesiology testing on pages xvii-xviii in the Introduction. Drink a glass of water and be certain that your environment is comfortable and peaceful. Sit in a comfortable chair for doing your self-testing. Have your 3x5 cards easily accessible to you, but be sure to turn the cards facedown before you begin testing.
- Sit in a comfortable and sturdy chair.
- Remember to maintain a neutral state of mind.
- Perform an "indicator muscle test" to determine your baseline strength by pushing on your dominant arm with your other hand. If you can easily resist moderate pressure, rest and then proceed.
- Take one 3x5 card and place it in your pocket or on your lap and then test this activity for compatibility in the same format as you used for the indicator muscle test.
    - If your body responds with a "strong" muscle test, you know that the potential activity or endeavor is compatible with your inner being.
    - If you find a "weak" muscle test, your arm is easily pushed downward, you are probably not currently compatible with the potential activity or new endeavor.

Use Your Mind
In recent decades the mind-body connection has been publicly disclosed and well documented. Athletic performance, for example, is bolstered by "pre-living" the sporting event. Some professional golfers will *think about* the golf course and its idiosyncrasies in vivid detail days and weeks in advance of their tournaments. The golfer then visualizes himself/herself performing optimally as they mentally plan their strategy. This may include setting up, swinging and achieving a stellar outcome at each of the course's holes.

Whether an athlete, artist or performer, those who can analyze their own strengths and weaknesses gain a much deeper understanding from that introspection, and then can more easily calibrate their performance or activity. They are often the ones who become champions and winners. This principle can also be applied to students of any subject, in preparing for exams and improving performance.

Becoming a top-notch "youthing expert"—a maturing adult who is committed to achieving vibrant health, happiness and wellbeing for themselves and others—can be analogous to becoming a winning pro-golfer. Success in any area rarely happens by accident. Instead, it involves careful planning and effort. You can both design your own plan to support healthy youthing and visualize its fulfillment. This book will be your guide in the process. In this way you too can become as successful in that arena as any professional athlete or acclaimed artist is in their field.

Begin Carving Your Niche *Now*
The list below contains many attitudes, ideals and behaviors that characterize a youthing potential. Women and men who live by and practice these methods are generally happier, healthier and are respected by others. Consider creating new vistas (goals or aims) of self-mastery for yourself, or affirming those you already have. This list will help you to remember your highest ideals, and encourage you to confidently move forward in your life.

Becoming Your Family's Matriarch or Patriarch
As you are carving your respected elder niche, you may (in a secular sense) be on the path to becoming your family's matriarch or patriarch (or patriarch/matriarch team). Many families gravitate toward having a matriarch, a patriarch or a team of respected and venerated elders who can and do set the tone for family interactions, values and celebrations. Today, each family and each individual in the family may have a distinct concept and way of relating to this respected elder position.

Well-established, elder-venerating traditions practiced for centuries are rapidly changing. In our time, we must accept that established traditions do not necessarily prevail, and realize that it is up to each of

> **How to Build and Manifest Your Own "Respected Elder" Niche**
> - Work to achieve your highest level of human potential.
> - Mindfully engage yourself in everything you do.
> - Enrich your life by pursuing worthy goals that you may not have had time for in the past. Now is the time to declare your life's passions and wholeheartedly pursue them.
> - Define your legacy; bequeath this legacy to your loved ones, family, community, or even humankind as a whole.
> - Determine how you can create a better world for future generations, and take action.
> - Create depth in your relationships, new and old alike. This includes mending misunderstandings or hurtful episodes.
> - Right your wrongs and be right with the world. (Ask for and gracefully receive forgiveness for mistakes, errors, and hurtful episodes that have occurred during your life.)
> - Live your life with intention (like you mean it).
> - Find more ways to contribute to the "greater good."
> - Actively move forward on your chosen spiritual path.
> - Live in gratitude daily.
> - Give and receive unconditional love unabashedly.
> - Seek help from others whose wisdom you respect to become truly effective in actualizing these steps.
> - Prepare to be a wise consultant for those who seek your insights and wisdom.

us to bring the best we can to the family dynamic, and to move forward toward our life goals. We are likely teaching by example. Are we seen as kind and compassionate individuals? Do we teach our grandchildren the art of critical thinking and judicious decision making by our examples? Are we passing on family traditions, lore, even recipes, etc. to the younger generations in our families? Spending the time to share sacred familial customs can be very enjoyable for you and instructive to those you are sharing with.

A healthful and balanced state of being for anyone includes being comfortable with one's age (whether it is stated in two digits or three). Hopefully, you have several intriguing new activities or "challenges" to pursue that can enrich yourself, and also your family and friends. Do not buy into the stereotyping of elderhood as being riddled with health problems and limitations. Certainly, as we accumulate years, we may also accumulate aches, pains and sometimes degrees of disability. This is a natural consequence of life. But, we can still embrace our status as capable and wise elders. Taking steps to improve your health and to enrich your life as you mature is possible for any individual regardless of age or ability. Now is the time to personalize your plan for creating the best "you" ever known to the world. Plan for a high level of health and wellness in your fulfilled life. Carve your niche! Keep enriching yourself and working to leave your mark today!

Clinical Kinesiology is and will be a useful tool to help you in these and other areas of your life.

LEARN MORE

Books

Child, Julia and Alex Prud'homme. *My Life in France*. New York: Anchor Books, 2007.

Grandma Moses and Otto Kallir. *Grandma Moses: My Life's History*. New York: Harper & Brothers, 1952.

Ingalls Wilder, Laura and Pamela Smith Hill. *Pioneer Girl: The Annotated Autobiography*. Pierre, South Dakota: South Dakota Historical Society Press, 2014

Lipton, Bruce H. *The Biology of Belief* 10th Anniversary Edition: *Unleashing the Power of Consciousness, Matter, & Miracles*. Carlsbad, Calif.: Hay House, 2015.

Montgomery, Ben. *Grandma Gatewood's Walk*. Chicago: Chicago Review Press, 2014.

Websites

www.familysearch.org
www.superseniors.org

CHAPTER 3

Coming to Terms

As we move forward in our journey toward and through elderhood, we each face personal and unique challenges. This chapter will assist you in coming to terms with these challenges, limitations and perceived obstacles. Hopefully, as the stories in this chapter indicate, you too will be balanced and resourceful as you learn to adapt to the obligatory changes nature provides. Coming to terms and creatively moving forward is rewarding and helps us prepare for new experiences.

Alyssa Mae had been my patient off and on for many years. After reaching her sixties, she frequently came to my office in the summer for back pain that always seemed to occur after her spring and summer garden planting. We talked about ways to minimize the strain on her back, and she modified her lifestyle a bit, but still habitually overworked her lower back. Eventually, after three or four painful gardening seasons, Alyssa Mae decided to start using raised gardens. She consulted with me about the potential design for these, and we utilized Clinical Kinesiology testing to determine the best height for the structures. We tested several potential heights for the raised beds, in 2-inch increments, and found that a height of 30 inches (76.2 centimeters) was the best option. The design also included garden seats that allowed her to rest and admire her handiwork.

As a few more years passed, Alyssa Mae found it difficult to drive confidently. Her vision slowly became dim and her depth perception dwindled. One day, she came to my office for treatment and announced that she was going to stop driving and give her car to her granddaughter. This was a thoughtful decision that she was comfortable making for herself. She knew that she could call upon friends and family for transportation or use a taxi if no one was available to help her on certain days. Because Alyssa Mae had given careful consideration to the pros, cons and alternatives, she was able to easily let go of her perceived notion that her independence was contingent on her ability to drive.

Ultimately, this decision to stop driving opened some new doors for her. Sally, Alyssa Mae's gardening friend, offered to take her to the local garden center to purchase her yearly supply of seedlings. Later, Sally invited her to join a local gardening club. The result was that Alyssa Mae met several new friends and included more meaningful activities into her life.

Twelve years later Alyssa Mae suffered a mild stroke that slowed her down both physically and mentally. For quite a few months various family members and friends helped her with her household chores, meal preparations, and a variety of other small tasks. Alyssa Mae faithfully maintained healthful lifestyle practices, wise food choices, and participated in physical therapy and a home exercise program.

After several months on this program, she had reached a therapeutic plateau. It became obvious that her need for a walker to safely navigate around her home, and on her outings, would be a permanent requirement. Since she had a large backyard, and her raised beds were quite a distance from her back door, she made the decision to discontinue her vegetable gardening. She asked her daughters to fill the raised beds with colorful annual flowers that she could see from her porch. Again, Alyssa Mae evaluated her situation and made thoughtful changes to her lifestyle. These changes took into consideration her safety, her preferences, and her love of aesthetic beauty. Her attitude and her thoughtful choices became an inspiration to many.

About two years after her stroke, Alyssa Mae reevaluated her life again. She found that her three-bedroom home and large yards contained more space and required more upkeep than she could adequately care for or fully enjoy. She and her family searched out independent living communities and located several potential candidates. Visiting each of these communities with her family, she had her photograph taken in each of her two favorite facilities. She then brought the photographs to one of her appointments with me. When she lay down on my treatment table, she began talking about her impressions of the first facility while looking at the photograph of herself inside the available apartment. We asked questions verbally, such as, "Is this new location compatible with my energy field?" Her muscle response was a strong YES. We tested the second location in a similar fashion, and found her muscle test yielded a weaker response. I explained that using Clinical Kinesiology for guidance in decision-making is helpful and should be considered along with many other relevant pieces of information. Alyssa Mae thanked me and told me that it was a comfort to have testing of this sort done. It confirmed her intuitive sense about the first apartment choice. When she and her family visited both venues once more, she was able to confidently select her preferred apartment, one that had been confirmed with muscle testing during our appointment.

Alyssa Mae sold her home and moved into a beautiful apartment in her favorite independent living community. The facility she chose was filled with friendly residents and it accommodated those who required walkers or wheelchairs. Lush outdoor gardens and beautiful indoor plants satisfied her inner gardener. The community had a restaurant, a small in-house theater, and multiple activity rooms for the residents. Her friend Sally liked the facility so well that she also moved into an apartment there.

These small vignettes of Alyssa Mae's life and her choices may be inspirational to anyone faced with making necessary lifestyle choices. After any significant change in life, we can decide to move forward and to take responsibility for this new current status instead of bemoaning the changes. In facing several dramatic life changes, Alyssa Mae coped well, used excellent discernment, and made life-enhancing and life-simplifying choices. While each situation was different, her attitude and honest assessment of her abilities were her saving graces, and resulted in a happy, life-enhancing environment. We all have more or less ability to do the same. Starting now, we can make important, positive, and healthful choices in our lives—whether they are seemingly minor or more dramatic in nature.

From Infancy On

We began to come to terms with growing older when we were infants. In fact, each growth and developmental stage represents our accommodation to growing older. We could look at this phenomenon simply with respect to our shoes and foot coverings. As a newborn, perhaps your parents placed tiny hand-knitted socks on your feet to keep them warm. By the time you were beginning to take steps and toddle, you were likely wearing your first pair of infant shoes. At four or five years old, you were probably running almost everywhere that you traveled, and you wore lace-up sport or athletic-styled shoes. In subsequent years, if you were involved in specific sports or activities, you accommodated your needs by having soccer cleats, hiking boots, ski boots, horseback riding boots, or ballet slippers. Making changes of equipment and shoes for various activities or stages of your development were both necessary and beneficial. In the same way, we will hopefully be "changing shoes" attentively throughout life, equipping ourselves well for each new activity, each new challenge.

Generally speaking, most people glide from one developmental life change to the next with brief planning and little reservation during their younger years and the years of growth and development. During our older years, however, some of us may need to make intentional new accommodations to assist our mobility. For some people, these may include adding orthotics to our shoes to give more arch support and stability, or finding specialized shoes that aid in balance. Health conditions, injuries and certain disabilities may require you to use a knee brace, cane, walker, or some other type of assistance for comfort and safety. If you require help of this nature, even in the short term, you may struggle a bit in coming to terms with your needs. By "reframing" your new need (giving a new or slightly different spin to your situation) as a potential benefit for your safety and function, or even comfort, you can then move forward with inner peace to integrate the necessary change into your life.

High-Elevation Hikers

Maria and Walter loved hiking at high elevations in the Rocky Mountains. For decades their favorite weekend activity was to hike well above the timberline. Often, they backpacked into the wilderness, hiking for several miles on Saturday, set up camp for the night, and then hiked to the top of a 13,000- or 14,000-foot mountain on Sunday morning. As they aged, and over a period of years, they slowly began to shorten these trips so that they could sleep in their own comfortable bed at night. I met Maria and Walter when they were both beyond eighty-two.

Maria talked of their decades of high-elevation hiking and was a bit nostalgic as she explained that neither of them was comfortable hiking over 9500 feet any longer. However, she quickly brought herself back to the present and said, "You know we have both been blessed to have been able to be so physically active for so many years, but now we are really enjoying being home on weekends and entertaining our grandchildren. They are the next generation of high-mountain hikers and I can encourage them and share our photographs and videos with them. I expect that my grandchildren will be more concertedly trekking the high mountain trails in the next few years."

Both Walter and Maria had been observant and had used field guide books during their hiking years. These books were a source of pleasure and education that gave them expertise in identifying many native plants. As their hiking hobby slowed, they decided to volunteer at the local nature center and ultimately guided groups of schoolchildren through wooded state parks, teaching them about the native plants and animals along the way. Occasionally, to their delight, some of their own grandchildren were able to join. Maria and Walter were able to utilize their nature skills and knowledge in a new way that ultimately benefited many other people. This was an excellent way to come to terms with their changing degree of physical abilities while maintaining contact with their beloved outdoors.

Another creative choice for many outdoor lovers has been to pull out a canvas and paints and render a lasting image of their favorite mountain scene or landscape. Others have used a simple sketchpad, brought a pen and poetry journal or carried a small musical instrument, like a recorder, on their hikes. In the process of painting, writing or playing music, the artist relives and celebrates his or her previous experiences. With your camera, pad and pencil, or canvas and brush, it is possible to preserve the beauty of a favorite spot for years to come.

Be Your Own CEO

Hopefully, each of us will have the courage and wherewithal to be the CEO of our own lives. Diligently learning about health-promoting diets, lifestyles, activities, thinking processes, and longevity-promoting measures *now,* empowers and moves you into a positive direction. Remembering to honor and update your life's purpose (*ikigai*)[1], sort of like your personal corporate mission statement, truly helps strengthen the fiber of your life and keeps you in that important, metaphoric CEO position for years to come.

A wise and proactive CEO will observe market conditions and current trends, and pay attention to their "gut feelings" to remain on the cutting edge of decision-making. These skills need very little translation to apply to running one's life. We might need to substitute "what do I *really* need?" or "what are my next anticipated needs?" for the terms "market conditions" and "current trends." Anticipating likely needs and changes *before* they are absolutely mandatory helps keep any personal CEO responsibly in charge and moving forward.

Unexpected circumstances, injuries, traumas and health conditions may crop up and divert or displace any of us from our CEO position. Plan B, which involves having a designated substitute, such as someone with medical power of attorney and/or durable power of attorney authority, is in the category of thoughtful pre-planning. Hopefully, most of us will not have a need for this type of substitute, but having the paperwork in order (even if we do not ultimately need it) can provide comfort. Obviously the best Plan A for any forward-thinking CEO is the plan to carry on effectively. Plan B, however, can be filed away for safekeeping.

The Best Part of Coming to Terms with Growing Older

Feeling gratitude about the gift of your life thus far, and cultivating hopeful prospects about your life experiences yet to come, is one of the best parts of elderhood. When we take time to reminisce as a means to feel the gratitude we may have originally skipped over, we are typically blessed with happiness and fulfillment. In general, gratitude begets happiness.

How sad to hurry without savoring these gifts of the older years. If you have hurried the past, work to recapture experiences, joyful events, triumphs, moments of true connection with loved ones, and live or relive the gratitude that you may have forgotten or skipped over. If you have been holding onto memories of events that moved you to feel slighted, let down, betrayed, or hurt, it is time to let go of your "negative charge" about those events. Now is the time to fill your memory with more positive and beneficial treasures. This action alone could elevate your mood and promote better brain function.

Gratitude: A New Habit

Acknowledging your blessings frequently is a wonderful way to move yourself forward with greater happiness and greater satisfaction with life. A number of research studies have demonstrated the benefits of expressing gratitude. Higher levels of wellness, true concern for others, optimism and even more restful sleep have been noted amongst people who use a Gratitude Journal. The studies have also shown diminished occurrences of depression, colds, substance abuse and various bothersome symptoms (aches, pains, headaches and digestive disturbances). It behooves all of us to begin recording our blessings in a Gratitude Journal.

You can do your recording in a very simple format on a calendar or in a spiral notebook, or you may choose to buy a bound journal. You can use this notebook/journal to reflect upon your day's thoughts and experiences in the evening, sometime before bed. Another approach is to make notes in your journal or on your calendar throughout the day as events you are grateful for take place. The action of reviewing your blessings and frequently reminding yourself of what you are thankful for is a critical part of this process. Some people prefer to make entries into their Gratitude Journal on a daily basis, while others prefer to journal one-to-three times each week. Since good habits are best established with daily repetition, I recommend that you concertedly work on your Gratitude Journal on a daily basis for at least twenty-one days, and then evaluate to determine if that level of consistency is something you can comfortably continue.

We are probably subconsciously thankful for many simple aspects of our lives that we seem to take for granted. Once we remember to acknowledge gratefulness for being alive, or having a wonderful "significant other," and supportive friends, and an astute mind, or a loyal pet, and a comfortable home, and the wherewithal to choose a path for a more enjoyable and richer future, we certainly become more focused on the positive gifts in our lives. These simple examples could be a starting point for your Gratitude Journal.

You may also want to create a preface to your Journal in which you list some of your blessings. Refer frequently to your list, perhaps with every writing session. Take time to reflect on these most precious gifts and acknowledge your gratitude for them.

You will be most successful if you can specifically describe aspects of your day, your life and your blessings. What are you most thankful for today? Weeks or months later, when you decide to look back at your entries for any certain date, you may smile or chuckle as you relive the fun or heartwarming event that you wrote about. An example of this could be your responses to your grandchild's first steps and the excitement and pride expressed by all who witnessed them. If you are able to add a photograph or hand-drawn sketch into your journal, it will be more engaging when you look back on it.

If you are recovering from an injury or a surgery, you can journal about your recovery mileposts, such as: *Monday. I am grateful that I was able to walk the length of the hall four times.* Followed by an entry a few days later: *Thursday. I am grateful that I was able to walk to the neighbor's house and back, and feel good.* And later that afternoon another entry: *I am so grateful that my friend came for a surprise lunch visit and she remembered that I love avocado and pine nuts on my salad!*

Months later, you may have recovered fully from your knee replacement, for instance, but may be struggling with your mood, the weather or a troubling issue. Simply looking back at your Gratitude Journal to recall the joy and pleasure of your many recorded experiences will raise your spirits again.

If you are having difficulty creating your Gratitude Journal, or even find yourself rehashing a list of hurtful or negative events, I suggest that you consult a Clinical Kinesiology practitioner to help you evaluate any trapped and/or stale bitterness and resentment. However, you may feel confident enough to proceed with self-testing first to define trapped emotions. Processing and then releasing these emotions will bring relief and lightness throughout your entire being.

Way of the Wise: The Path of Forgiveness
Throughout our lifetime each of us undoubtedly has many opportunities to forgive. Not taking the opportunity, or postponing it, impedes our inner wellbeing, and our ability to smoothly interact with others. Opportunities to forgive may include situations between yourself and childhood playmates, siblings, pets, parents, children, colleagues, significant others, yourself or even your Creator. Starting early in life to practice forgiveness will help foster better communication and deeper relationship connections throughout your life. If you have missed taking advantage of forgiveness opportunities, now is the time to rectify that.

Forgiveness promotes your own equanimity, inner peace and happiness. When you practice forgiveness you are freeing yourself of emotional baggage. Once you have given yourself a chance to process your grief and hurt feelings and have consciously decided to forgive, you will be abundantly blessed by a new sense of ease in your life.

When you are processing a grievance and preparing to forgive the perpetrator, who may have unknowingly committed what you consider to be an affront or damaging action, you may actually need to experience and wrestle with one or several of the five stages of grief. These stages, researched and defined by Elisabeth Kübler-Ross are: 1. denial, 2. anger, 3. bargaining, 4. depression, and 5. acceptance. After any sort of loss, injury, or grief-worthy scenario, all human beings tend to experience and move through these emotional stages at their own individualized pace, but not necessarily in a clear-cut order.

By the time you consciously decide to forgive, you may have already moved through the first stage or two of the grieving process (denial, anger). Removing self-imposed blockages, such as anger and vengeance, and moving through the natural progression of stages 1 through 5 will prepare you to actually and wholeheartedly forgive. If you feel stuck or blocked, as many people do, know that this is a very human experience, and a good time to seek assistance. Speaking to a close friend with whom you can comfortably share such personal challenges may be sufficient. Consulting a professional therapist, counselor, psychologist, clergy member, or Clinical Kinesiologist may be even more beneficial. This guidance could help you "see the forest" in spite of the trees, to sort out your pain and your response to that pain. A competent professional will also be able to assure you that your struggle is comparable to many others' experiences, and *can* be resolved.

The 18th-century English poet Alexander Pope wrote, "To err is human, to forgive divine." This includes cases of you hurting others in some fashion. Often the injured person becomes stunned or shut down enough that they have difficulty bouncing back to optimal function. Anger and resentment are natural defense mechanisms that have purpose in the short-term, but become real hindrances to your emotional wellbeing if allowed to become long-term aspects of your psyche.

Sometimes we have the greatest difficulty forgiving ourselves for mistakes, errors, poor judgment, or instances where we've inflicted pain on ourselves or others. We all deserve a proper apology and ultimate acceptance *from ourselves*. Learning to be loving and gracious to ourselves can be a template for being forgiving and accepting of others. You can begin to spread this loving approach by forgiving yourself for your mistakes, misdeeds and bad decisions. Then, move on to forgiving others for their infractions. You may need to *practice* forgiveness several times before attempting to forgive deeply wounding transgressions. You can forgive the person for their wrongdoing, and not condone or excuse the hurtful act. This will reduce stress and increase peace in your life.

If you have trepidations about opening an old "wound" that you have not forgiven, seek counsel. Think of this as having a surgeon's help when an old, festering wound is abscessing and needs to be lanced, drained and bandaged. The momentary pain is well worth enduring in order to gain the ultimate healing.

If you have hurt or offended someone, or even more seriously compromised someone, attempt to gain their forgiveness. Your first step may be to closely consider the event or situation and consider what the other person must have experienced and felt. Try your best to get in touch with your compassionate nature. The next step will be to apologize in earnest, whether in person, or by a written message. This is the part of the process that is under your control. The other person will decide to forgive you or not. In either case, you have put forth your sincerest effort and likely will have a good measure of relief about the situation.

Whether you give or receive forgiveness, the result is a more open heart, a more peaceful mind and a readiness for healing—physiological, emotional and spiritual. Actively forgiving and releasing pain and resentment will free you to more actively live in gratitude and compassion. Realize that withholding forgiveness reinforces your role as a victim and energetically allows the offender to continue to wield some power and control over you. Once you have consciously and with wholehearted intention forgiven someone, you are no longer a victim of their wrongdoing. You may be able to have a new understanding or sense of compassion for your offender. More likely, you will have increased compassion and awareness about the fragility of the human psyche.

Research shows that people who practice forgiveness experience many physical and emotional health benefits.

Forgiveness Can Lead to:
- Healthier relationships
- Greater spiritual and psychological wellbeing
- Less anxiety, stress and hostility
- Lower blood pressure
- Fewer symptoms of depression
- Stronger immune system
- Improved heart health
- Higher self-esteem.[2]

Each event deserving of your forgiveness is unique and will require its own processing time. If you are new to the concept of consciously and concertedly forgiving, you will be amazed at the benefits you reap.

Choose Elder Terms Wisely

Your choice of language—words and phrases—is of utmost importance. This is especially true of your body's inner language, which you are beginning to understand through Clinical Kinesiology. The words you choose to use in your everyday life set the tone for your mood, impact your self-esteem and shape your reality.

The descriptive language used by media and society in general to depict the aging population is often less than favorable. Whether you intend to or not, you are influenced by this language and may sometimes adopt these depreciating words and ideas as your own truth.

Older populations, especially in the Westernized world, are often portrayed as "grumpy old fogies," incompetent and burdensome individuals, and even mentally inept. We are inundated with these unfair and essentially incorrect concepts of what it means to be an aging person. You must be diligent to observe them, and not identify with these concepts that can actively creep into your psyche and infiltrate your reality.

Begin by examining your own beliefs around aging, and your expectations of elderhood, in order to scrutinize your personal fears and discomforts. I invite you to courageously make a list of the words and phrases you hear or know of that reinforce these negative views. Consider each of these concepts so that you can begin to really explore your personal beliefs about becoming older. If you sit with these ideas even briefly, you will recognize their falsities. You will quickly begin to see that you are not a "grumpy old geezer," a "crazy, blue-haired old lady," an inept burden, or any of the other negative stereotypes you may have been exposed to, or even adopted. Once the list is compiled and considered, throw it away, literally and figuratively. From that moment forward, commit to noticing and dissolving these negative images and ideas from your psyche. They will not disappear entirely, but as you observe them you can assert, "I no longer choose to accept … as applying to myself." Also re-commit to not using them in speaking to or about yourself or others.

Next I recommend that you make a list of the wonderful things you are: A wise elder, your family's historian, a living library of knowledge, a most blessed individual that has been afforded the miracle of life's many stages, etc. You will soon begin to see that you are not congruent with the stereotypes portrayed in the media or the depressing picture depicted by society. If you catch yourself reverting back to the negative ideas of elderhood, quickly remember to replace them with images of all the positive things that you *really* are. Keep this positive list and refer back to it often. Remind yourself of the magnificent person you are. You are wise, experienced and insightful. Many of the wonderful characteristics you possess come from your awesome transformation into elderhood.

As you clear cobwebs out of your emotional self and begin to both feel and express gratitude and forgiveness, you will be much more at ease in your life. As you continue to practice the recommendations in this chapter, you will find that coming to terms with changes and obstacles in your path gradually becomes more second nature. From this fresh and even exhilarating vantage point, you can feel and express compassion for others, as well as for yourself, and be more successful at coming to terms with any challenge you face.

Moving away from a sedentary lifestyle and incorporating purposeful activity is a well documented and viable way to enhance your life.[3] The next chapter efficiently brings this information to you.

LEARN MORE
Review Chapter 3, "Energy and Emotions" in *Your Body Can Talk, 2nd Edition* by Susan L. Levy, D.C. for more guidance on proactively clearing and rebalancing your emotional self.

Books
Arrien, Angeles. *Living in Gratitude: Mastering the Art of Giving Thanks Every Day, A Month-By-Month Guide.* Boulder, Colo.: Sounds True, Inc., 2001.
DeMoss, Nancy Leigh. *Choosing Gratitude: Your Journey to Joy.* Chicago: Moody Publishers, 2011.
Dowling Singh, Kathleen. *The Grace in Aging: Awaken as You Grow Older.* Somerville, Mass.: Wisdom Publications, 2014.

Hawkins, David R., M.D., Ph.D. *Letting Go: The Pathway of Surrender.* Carlsbad, Calif.: Hay House, 2014.

Kübler-Ross, Elisabeth. *On Death and Dying: What the Dying Have to Teach Doctors, Nurses, Clergy and Their Own Families, Scribner Trade Paperback Edition.* New York: Scribner, 2014.

Kushner, Harold, S. *When Bad Things Happen to Good People.* New York: Anchor Books, 2004.

Richmond, Lewis. *Aging as a Spiritual Practice: A Contemplative Guide to Growing Older.* New York: Avery Publishing, 2012.

Ryan, M.J. *Attitudes of Gratitude: How to Give and Receive Joy Everyday of Your Life.* York Beach, Maine: Conari Press, 1999

Schachter-Shalomi, Zalman and Ronald S. Miller. *From Age-ing to Sage-ing: A Revolutionary Approach to Growing Older.* New York: Grand Central Publishing, 2014.

Shelton, Charles M. Ph.D. *The Gratitude Factor: Enhancing Your Life through Grateful Living.* Yonkers, New York: Hidden Spring Press, 2010.

Smedes, Lewis B. *Forgive and Forget: Healing the Hurts We Don't Deserve.* San Francisco: HarperOne, 2007.

Vanzant, Iyanla. *Forgiveness: 21 Days to Forgive Everyone for Everything.* Carlsbad, Calif.: Smiley Books, 2013.

Viorst, Judith. *Necessary Losses: The Loves, Illusions, Dependencies, and Impossible Expectations That All of Us Have to Give Up in Order to Grow.* New York: Fireside: 1998.

Endnotes, Chapter 3

1. Tanno, Kozo, Kiyomi Sakataa , Masaki Ohsawaa, Toshiyuki Onodaa , Kazuyoshi Itaia , Yumi Yaegashia and Akiko Tamakoshib. "Associations Of Ikigai as a Positive Psychological Factor with All-Cause Mortality And Cause-Specific Mortality Among Middle-Aged and Elderly Japanese People: Findings from the Japan Collaborative Cohort Study." *Journal of Psychosomatic Research*, 67 (2009), 67-75.

2. Mayo Clinic Staff. "Forgiveness: Letting Go of Grudges and Bitterness." Mayo Clinic: November 11, 2014. http://www.mayoclinic.org/healthy-lifestyle/adult-health/in-depth/forgiveness/art-20047692

3. Kirk-Sanchez, Neva J. and Ellen L. McGough. "Physical Exercise and Cognitive Performance in the Elderly: Current Perspectives." *Clinical Interventions in Aging*, 9 (2014), 51-62.

CHAPTER 4

Move It and Preserve It

"Move it" pertains to moving your body. On a daily basis, purposely putting intentional movement (such as frequent standing, walking up stairs rather than using an elevator, weeding a garden) into your regimen can be as beneficial as thirty to sixty minutes dedicated to exercise. Thinking of new ways to engage in purposeful movement will be a great help in your body's health and your overall wellbeing.

Your body was designed to be in almost constant motion. Even during sleep we move—tossing, turning and twitching. These are examples of our larger muscles moving during sleep. In fact, researchers have documented that we all burn a certain amount of calories with each hour of sleep. This amount varies depending on a person's weight, temperature and movement patterns. Of course, our heart, circulatory system, lungs, kidneys and gastrointestinal system are continuously performing needed functions, while at the same time purposefully moving. In fact, movement has been considered a qualification for determining whether an organism is alive.

Joan Vernikos, Ph.D., as the director of NASA's life sciences division for thirty years, studied the effects of Gravitational Deprivation Syndrome on American astronauts during their time in space. She shares conclusive evidence about the requirement for continuous movement by human beings. In her book *Sitting Kills Moving Heals,* Vernikos writes:

> *It turns out that the best technique [for delaying physical deterioration] is quite different from the common method of*

exercising in a gym once a day or several times a week. Rather, a multitude of frequent, low-intensity stimuli, throughout the day, 365 days a year is the optimal approach. In other words, the secret to good health on earth that space exploration revealed is the need for perpetual motion.[1]

One of Vernikos' most important recommendations is for people to change positions frequently. For those who sit at work or those who sit during leisure time, she suggests standing up for several minutes, walking or engaging in some other movement for several minutes twice per hour. An example of purposeful movement at work is standing up from your workstation and walking to the water cooler or kitchen to get a drink of water (drink heartily to flush your system, and induce a new excuse to get up and walk to the bathroom). Another example is walking to a printer, wastebasket or other necessary work area that you purposely place at a distance to encourage purposeful movement into your workday.

Some forward-looking companies have ergonomic and health-orientated office plans that include designated walking paths so that people can actually walk laps around their offices, even while having brief meetings with colleagues, either in person or by telephone. A new and growing trend for the office environment is to utilize standing desks and/or treadmill desks. New workspaces are being designed so that the individual can sit, stand or be on a treadmill and alternate these positions and activities throughout the day. Not only allowing, but encouraging movement in the workplace diminishes incidences of neck pain, back pain and afternoon sluggishness, and boosts productivity. If you are fortunate enough to work in an office that has integrated some of these procedures, you are not as likely to be fatigued or mentally burned out at the end of your workday. If you are not in such an environment, you can be proactive in implementing some of these purposeful activities for yourself.

Vernikos also found that non-astronauts who lead sedentary lifestyles, sitting many hours per day, become vulnerable to the same Gravity Deprivation Syndrome symptoms that plague many astronauts.

Some astronauts are able to quickly recover from these symptoms once they land back on Earth and resume normal activity, but for certain individuals, especially those who go on longer space missions, the recovery time is surprisingly prolonged.

> **A Partial List of Signs and Symptoms of Being Sedentary**
> - Poor Posture
> - Diminished Lung Capacity
> - Reduced Bone Density
> - Reduced Muscle Mass
> - Lack of Muscle Strength
> - Flabbiness of the Muscles
> - Decreased Efficiency of the Heart
> - Hormonal Imbalances
> - Joint Pain
> - Sluggish Digestion

While packing up a duffel bag and moving through traffic to squeeze time in at the gym may work for many people, the process dissuades many would-be gym goers who simply go home and plop down on their couches. If you are successful at maintaining a good pattern of gym or other sport or exercise activities, by all means continue. If not, Dr. Vernikos and others advocate that, for the majority of people, simply weaving movement into the fabric of your daily life may be more realistic, cost-effective and palatable.

It is possible to play at this work of adding movement. When going grocery shopping, look for a distant parking space to increase your moments of walking between your car and the store. When you come home, you may choose to increase the distance that you carry the grocery bags by walking around the house to a different door. You can also integrate movement and exercise into your routine by unloading heavier items and setting them on the particular shelf in sets of three or five repetitions. When doing laundry, you might consider an outdoor clothesline that will save fuel, increase your activity, and provide fresher-smelling laundry. A useful step is to consider daily tasks and chores as beneficial movement or even play. Your mental attitude and your physical body benefit immensely from this.

When you take a break from sitting, you might turn on music and dance. You can also dance while folding your clean fresh laundry, or dance a little bit during food preparation in the kitchen. What ideas do you have for including movement and having fun at the same time? The possibilities are practically endless.

Non-Exercise Activity Thermogenesis (NEAT)
The term *thermogenesis* was coined by the forward-thinking doctor, James A. Levine, M.D. Dr. Levine has studied movement versus being sedentary, noting the various health implications of each. He describes his research in his book *Get Up!* Dr. Levine reports that the average walking speed for people is 1.1 mph. He also discovered that obese people typically sit at least two hours and fifteen minutes more each day than lean people.[2] One of Dr. Levine's greatest accomplishments was to assist in the development of movement-oriented school environments that resulted in better learning environments, lower stress for students, and a reduction of hyperactivity in movement-deprived children. He was the inventor (in 2000) of the "Treadmill Task." Based on his work, numerous companies now produce a variety of treadmill desks that provide exercise, purposeful activity, stress reduction, and improved productivity for their users.

Dr. Levine is a great proponent of non-exercise activity thermogenesis (NEAT), and encourages people to simply add purposeful movement throughout each day. He also developed a variety of movement-sensing or activity-tracking devices to be worn by laboratory animals and human beings. The data gathered from these sensors is described in his book and other works. Dr. Levine lectures and writes about the sitting disease that perpetuates obesity, heart disease, diabetes, some forms of cancer, depression, and numerous other health conditions. He presents a simple remedy: *Get Up!* out of your chair and find new ways and reasons to move. I suggest you read his book *Get Up!* for more information.

Tai Chi

Tai Chi, also known as Tai Chi Chuan, Taijiquan and Tai Chi Chih, is the most commonly practiced exercise/art form on Earth. This graceful and meditative martial art form was developed in medieval China. Tai Chi contains both philosophical and physical activity components. Modern-day research has correlated numerous health benefits, both physical and emotional, to the practice of Tai Chi and its related martial art form, Qi Gong. While these are two quite distinct disciplines, they have been categorized as one for the purposes of most research studies. To simplify our discussion, this book will refer to the benefits of both Tai Chi and Qi Gong simply as Tai Chi. You can easily access Tai Chi classes, videos and instruction in your local communities as well as online.

The ancient roots of Tai Chi, dating from approximately the twelfth century, are believed to emanate from a Taoist monastery. Zhang Sanfeng is the monk credited with its development. Over many centuries, Tai Chi has undergone modifications, and various masters have developed specific styles. Historically, there are only five forms of Tai Chi, each of which had specific applications developed between the late 1500s and the early 1900s. A more contemporary modification is called "easy Tai Chi" or "Tai Chi Chih." While these historical details are interesting, the important message overall is how beneficial, health promoting and youth preserving Tai Chi is!

Tai Chi is a grounding, dancelike, moving meditation. Numerous positions and poses are studied and then put together as a flowing sequence that balances your body, mind and even your spirit. The movements are slow, purposeful and often circular. As you are taught some of the positions, you may be asked to imagine, for instance, that you are holding a twelve- to fifteen-inch beach ball in front of you. You may then imagine that you are rotating this ball so that the right and left palms of your hands face each other and continue moving one above the other. You may then be instructed about matching your breathing to the movements, focusing and moving with a rhythmic pattern. Generally, in most Tai Chi practice, your feet are placed in a wide stance, one foot placed approximately the length of one foot in front of the other (your comfort and balance are more important than the actual distance). Often, you will shift your weight from the forward foot to the backward foot in a comfortable and easy rocking rhythm.

This foot placement instruction truly helps you balance your body physically and "ground" yourself to the earth. In fact, Tai Chi is traditionally practiced outdoors, often in a grassy field or park, wearing thin-soled shoes so that there is little impediment to the earth energy coming into your body. In this way, Tai Chi can facilitate "earthing," a process of energetic connecting to the earth. Practicing Tai Chi and spending minutes actively connecting to the earth with your bare, or almost bare, feet (earthing) may help you to balance your body and dissipate some of the traumatic effects of electromagnetic pollution. Modern research finds that elders who undertake Tai Chi commonly have improved balance after twenty sessions.[3] Other studies indicate that Tai Chi can also help elders overcome the fear of falling (Zhang, et al. 2006).[4]

Tai Chi Practice Therapeutically Benefits These Health Conditions

Total Body/General Symptoms
- Low energy
- Reduced stamina
- Poor balance
- Muscular weakness
- Diabetes
- Arthritis
- Pain
- Stiffness
- Osteoporosis
- Decreased immunity
- Poor sleep
- Lacking a sense of wellbeing
- Lacking a sense of connectedness or community

Respiratory System
- Shallow breathing

Skin Issues
- Susceptibility to shingles

Cardio-Vascular
- High blood pressure
- Heart failure
- Poor circulation
- Lymphatic congestion
- Atrial fibrillation

Nervous System (Brain, Mind and Emotions)
- Poor balance
- Decreased cognitive function
- Stress
- Depression
- Anxiety
- ADHD
- Neurodegenerative disorders
    - Alzheimer's
    - Multiple Sclerosis
    - Parkinson's

Gastro-Intestinal
- Digestive disturbances

Tai Chi is often practiced as a group endeavor and provides a nice opportunity for socialization. This aspect may contribute to Tai Chi's overall health-enhancing quality. Tai Chi offers physical benefit as a low impact aerobic activity, and may also increase brain volume and function, increase memory, and reduce the risk of Alzheimer's. There are so many good reasons to learn Tai Chi that I strongly encourage this practice, regardless of your chronological age.

Yoga

Historically, yoga (the word means "union") has been a philosophy, a way of life, and a cultural and a spiritual path. For our purposes here, we will focus essentially on *hatha yoga* (the movement, stretching, strengthening part) and *pranayama* (the breathing part), both of which greatly benefit any practitioner.

If you are already a yoga practitioner, please continue with your favorite yogic style. If you have not yet been a student or practitioner of yoga, do not wait another day. Yoga classes are easily found online, at recreation centers, at yoga schools and centers, or may even be available on your local public television station. Hatha yoga (as taught by the Iyengar school, among others) offers well-established methods that address the needs of a beginning yoga practitioner.

Hatha yoga's popularity is growing exponentially in the Western world today because of its profound effectiveness. There are now hatha yoga classes available for individuals with particular needs: prenatal yoga classes, rehabilitative yoga classes (for those recovering from injury or other health conditions), children's yoga and yoga for elders. Various yoga postures (*asanas*) are designed to specifically address particular bones, joints or muscles. You may want to refer to *The New Yoga for People over Fifty* by Suza Francina, RYT.

Yogic poses are generally categorized for beginners, intermediate practitioners, or advanced yoga practitioners. Proper instruction is essential for beginners, as is taking the time to listen to your own body "talk," as you personalize your own yogic practice. For instance, if you have had a joint replacement, surgery or a significant injury, it may not be advisable for you to perform certain asanas. If it is painful or problematic to achieve or maintain a particular pose, you are likely not yet ready for that particular asana. It may be wise to "under-challenge" yourself during your first several yoga sessions in order to avoid injury. As you become familiar with the practice of yoga and your body's abilities, you can safely and comfortably progress incrementally to more challenging poses.

Focusing on your breathing (pranayama), being in tune with your awareness, and beginning to meditate are integral to a general yogic practice. Some of the common benefits you may experience after yogic exercise include relaxation, stress reduction, improved mood and improved cognitive function. Since yoga means union, it is appropriate to say that yoga unites and coordinates your physical body, your mind and your entire being. Those who practice yoga reap physical, mental, emotional, and spiritual benefits. Yoga may be a path to greater balance in all aspects of your life.

The lists below contain fascinating and documented health benefits attributed to yoga.

> **Health Benefits of Yoga**
>
> *Structural System*
> - Improved and maintained bone density, integrity, and strength
> - Improved mobility
> - Improved posture (reversal of habitual slumped posture)
> - Increased and maintained muscle strength
> - Increased and maintained muscle tone
>
> *Heart and Cardiovascular System*
> - Lowering of high blood pressure
> - Lowering of high cholesterol
> - Reduced episodes of atrial fibrillation
> - Stabilized or normalized heart rhythms
>
> *Endocrine System*
> - Decreased insulin sensitivity
> - Diminished stress
> - Greater sense of calm
> - Improved mood
> - Improved sense of well-being
> - Increased low hormone functionality (melatonin, DHEA, and thyroid hormones)

Respiratory System
- Improved lung capacity

Mental/Emotional
- Diminished anxiety
- Diminished depression

Neurological
- Diminishment of tremors (Parkinson's and non-Parkinson's)
- Improved balance
- Improved coordination
- Improved posture

Cognitive Function
- Greater mental focus
- Improved attentiveness
- Improved critical thinking
- Improved language skills
- Improved problem-solving
- Increased ability to reason and make decisions

Essentrics

Essentrics is another amazing self-help movement methodology. It is based on a whole-body stretching technique developed by Miranda Esmonde-White, a former ballet dancer. Ms. Esmonde-White utilized principles from Tai Chi, ballet, stretching and muscle physiology to create this innovative method. In her book, *Aging Backwards: Reverse the Aging Process and Look 10 Years Younger in 30 Minutes a Day*, she explains the background philosophy and method of performance for the series of graceful, circular, full body stretches. The second half of her book is a pictorial guide to many stretches and workouts.

The author distinguishes between *concentric* and *eccentric* muscle movement. In brief, *concentric muscle movement* is utilized by weight trainers and those who do active competitive sports and running or track. Individuals involved in those sports frequently have injuries, which Esmonde-White believes are largely due to tight muscles that aren't able to stretch and relax. The epitome of concentric muscle movement would be doing multiple reps of biceps curls or squats with weights. This persistent contraction of the major muscle groups, which folds the muscle and brings it in closer to the torso, exemplifies concentric muscle contraction. In contrast, stretching while lengthening the major muscle groups and moving them away from the body's center exemplifies *eccentric muscle movement*. Esmonde-White writes:

> *Eccentric movement happens when a muscle extends and lengthens while in contraction. For example, when we lower a heavy bag of groceries, the elbow straightens and makes the biceps lengthen, creating an eccentric movement. Even though it is elongating as it lowers the heavy groceries, the biceps remains contracted.*[5]

The author, who has studied physiology and many varieties of exercise and fitness programs for years, weaves factual information from her studies throughout her book. She comes to some of the same conclusions that Joan Vernikos, Ph.D. and James A. Levine, M.D. do, concerning the benefits of near constant motion for humans. Esmonde-White is adamant that static (motionless) muscle contraction can be more harmful than beneficial. In Chapter 5, titled, "Stretch It Out: Flexibility Is the Fountain of Youth," she wisely proposes that if we properly stretch our muscles we relieve tension in the body, we allow all of the joints, both weight bearing and non-weight-bearing to function at best, and we improve our overall body function.

You may already have some difficulty bending down, walking or performing daily activities. For a moment, mentally contrast that stiff or painful feeling, that limited range of motion, with the sense of your muscles and joints being very relaxed and loose. It seems obvious that if you consistently work on healthful reasonable stretching, you can relieve, remedy or even avoid altogether those feelings of limitation, becoming more vibrantly involved in life and in your favorite activities.

Walking

The simplest movement and exercise activity for most people is walking. Anyone who has the physical ability to walk can benefit from purposely walking. Instead of simply walking from chair to couch or from a chair to your car, you can begin to consider walking as a life-giving, health-promoting form of exercise. For most of human existence, walking was not only the preferred, but the *only* means of transportation available to our ancestors. As various cultures have modernized, human walking has been minimized. For most people the actual facts concerning the beneficial qualities of walking have been left by the wayside as well.

You can undertake walking with a friend or loved one for companionship and an opportunity for uninterrupted communication if you so choose. Walking through the woods, a park, or any natural setting can engender relaxation, tranquility and peace of mind in addition to purposeful physical activity.

Simply walking for thirty-to-sixty minutes per day can improve your balance and agility measurably. Researchers have correlated the benefit of purposeful walking to a reduced risk of falling for elders. As well, the habit of walking correlates to reduced blood pressure and measurable stress reduction.

Dedicating thirty-to-sixty minutes of walking per day has been shown to balance metabolism, especially that of fats and carbohydrates. For some people, a good walking habit may help with reducing high blood sugar and also may reduce body fat. Since consistent walking can help your body's fat metabolism, it can also contribute to balancing your hormonal system. Obviously, if you have significant issues in these areas you will be well advised to consult your natural healthcare provider or medical provider to discuss your walking plan as a part of your entire health management program.

Many people find that walking helps clear their mind, helps them with their creativity, and helps calm their emotions, particularly after a stressful day or an upsetting event.

Of course, consistent walking will help tone your gluteus, thigh and calf muscles. You can expand the muscle-toning effect by engaging more muscles than would be strictly necessary for simple walking.

To make walking your exercise of choice simply include swinging or purposefully moving the arms, turning your head from side to side, and even adding some occasional sidesteps to call upon additional muscle groups.

Walking backwards is a self-care therapy for those with chronic low back pain, even lumbar disc problems. If you experiment with walking backwards, remember safety first. Begin with a familiar controlled environment, such as a hallway or room in your home that has been cleared of all tripping hazards. The first few times you engage in walking backwards it would be advisable to have a human spotter who would walk forward along with you, and would effectively be your "eyes," scouting out your path. If you become comfortable with this exercise you may graduate to using a hand-held mirror after having checked your path for tripping hazards.

Even if you have no chronic back pain, a brief stint of walking backwards can be a helpful brain and coordination stimulus. Some individuals experiencing Parkinson's symptoms find it easier to walk backwards than to walk forwards. They should be assisted to walk backwards as much as possible, for the therapeutic benefit. For the majority of people, walking backwards will be like a condiment added to their walking menu, not the main course.

Words of the Wise about Walking

In short, walking comes naturally to most of us, yet many simply have a daily walking deficiency. Hopefully you will find a few of the following quotes about walking to be inspirational. Perhaps you will consider writing a few yourself.

- Above all, do not lose your desire to walk. Every day I walk myself into a state of well-being and walk away from every illness. —Søren Kierkegaard

- An early-morning walk is a blessing for the whole day. —Henry David Thoreau

- We ought to take outdoor walks, to refresh and raise our spirits by deep breathing in the open air.—Lucius Annaeus Seneca

- Walking is also an ambulation of mind.—Gretel Ehrlich

- Walking is good for solving problems—it's like the feet are little psychiatrists.—Terri Guillemets

- One step at a time is good walking.—Chinese Proverb

- Thoughts come clearly while one walks.—Thomas Mann

- The best remedy for a short temper is a long walk.—Jacqueline Schiff

- After a day's walk everything has twice its usual value.—George Macauley Trevelyan

- Many people nowadays live in a series of interiors…disconnected from each other. On foot everything stays connected…—Rebecca Solnit

Chiropractic Care for Flexibility

An excellent way for you to ensure optimal joint function, mobility and range of motion is to seek chiropractic care from an experienced and trusted practitioner. Some chiropractors specialize in pediatrics, sports injury, geriatrics or other specific areas, but most chiropractors see a variety of patients and individualize their treatment style for each patient. In my own chiropractic practice, I have measured the available range of motion in an area of the body, such as the neck or lower back, before and after a patient's treatment, and seen a gain of ten to twenty degrees mobility in one treatment! Of course, results are often more gradual and consistent chiropractic treatment generally yields the best results.

Many professional and semi-professional athletes receive chiropractic treatment prior to games and sporting events and find noticeably improved performance. Once I was asked to treat a famous actress backstage with chiropractic care. She had fallen and injured her lower back during a rehearsal. I came to her performances with my portable treatment table, and treated her between each act on two consecutive nights. Her show did go on!

By far, the greatest benefit of chiropractic care is its balancing and normalizing effect on the nervous system. This allows for optimization of nerve supply to all organs, glands, muscles and bones. The result is a healthier, more durable, flexible and resilient body.

Many chiropractors are proficient in Applied Kinesiology and a smaller number are Clinical Kinesiologists. These dedicated natural healthcare professionals will also be able to test you via Kinesiology to gain answers to a vast array of your health related questions.

Other Movement Options

You may already enjoy or be involved in one or more physical activities that bring you pleasure or some sense of fulfillment. If you are comfortable with this activity and feel you tolerate it well, by all means continue. Some of these activities might include swimming, water aerobics, horseback riding, skiing, bicycling, tennis or dancing. Square dancing is particularly therapeutic in that you must process auditory input from the square dance caller and immediately translate that into your physical movement. I knew a wonderful ninety-three-year-old woman, who had been square dancing for decades and danced four or five nights each week until three months before her passing. She told me that square dancing is what "kept her going."

Richard, a friend of my editor, Regina Ryan, recently celebrated his eightieth birthday by completing an eighty-mile bike ride. He was so enthusiastic about bicycling that he scheduled three more eighty-mile bike rides during the following year.

Other movement activities to consider may include team sports such as volleyball, softball, basketball, etc. One of my friends and colleagues, Dr. William Koontz, is training to be part of a senior basketball team. The main requirements for this basketball team are that all members must be fit, agile and at least seventy years old!

Each of us needs to devise *A Move It and Preserve It* daily program of purposeful movement. Fortunately, we have a time-tested tool at our disposal to help us in designing a plan that is unique and useful to each of us. That tool is Clinical Kinesiology.

Move It and Preserve It, Basics

1. Minimize being sedentary, lessen your sitting time (if your physical condition allows)

2. Incorporate more physical activity and purposeful movement into your daily life within your home, apartment or office.

3. Explore a type of movement or stretching discipline that you can do simply at home. Great examples include Essentrics, yoga, and Tai Chi.

4. Continue or add enjoyable exercise or sports activities which you tolerate well.

5. Continue or begin chiropractic treatment to help with flexibility and health optimization.

If you have little or no experience with yoga or Tai Chi it would be best to take classes and receive sufficient instruction to feel comfortable doing the basics at home. Continuing in the class is also beneficial and allows for group involvement and interaction. You have many healthful options to choose from in designing your *Move it and Preserve It* program.

This system can help you determine which of these various activities are most compatible with your body and your inner self. Here's how:

1. Enroll the help of a professional, use a friend, or test yourself using the muscle-testing methods we've explained in this book.

2. Do a "trial run," that is, practice one movement activity (such as Tai Chi or walking) for a few minutes.

Move It and Preserve It   49

3. Then sit comfortably for a moment and muscle test yourself (or enlist the help of a friend or professional) asking (mentally or verbally) if your body and entire self feels compatible with this activity.

4. If your indicator muscle is strong during the test you can be assured that the activity is compatible with your body.

5. Also, test to ask yourself how often you should practice this discipline each week, or how long to participate in each session

6. Special Note: Within any particular exercise or movement discipline there may be certain postures or factors that are incompatible with your body's needs and abilities, and may cause pain or difficulty. If you have this experience, obviously eliminate any specific position or movement that causes pain or dysfunction in any part of your body.

7. If the results of your own muscle testing are confusing for you, or if you have reservations about a certain exercise or movement, avoid that particular exercise and seek counsel with your instructor, your Clinical Kinesiologist, or another healthcare practitioner. Generally speaking, the movement disciplines described in this chapter can be adapted to suit almost any individual. In fact, "sitting-only" versions of yoga (sometimes called Chair Yoga) and specially modified Tai Chi classes exist for those who need them.

Remember to keep moving to retain physical function and support your youthing lifestyle.

LEARN MORE
Review page 178 of *Your Body Can Talk, 2nd Edition* by Susan L. Levy, D.C. for more information on "earthing."

Books
Esmonde-White, Miranda. *Aging Backwards: Reverse the Aging Process and Look 10 Years Younger in 30 Minutes a Day.* New York: HarperCollins Books, 2014.

Francina, Suza RYT. *The New Yoga for People over Fifty*. New York: Health Communications, 1997.

Levine, James A. *Get Up!: Why Your Chair is Killing You and What You Can Do About It.* New York: St. Martin's Press LLC, 2014.

Montgomery, Ben. *Grandma Gatewood's Walk: The Inspiring Story of the Woman Who Saved the Appalachian Trail.* Chicago: Chicago Review Press, 2014.

Plasker, Eric, D.C.. *The 100 year Lifestyle: Dr. Plasker's Breakthrough Solution for Living Your Best Life—Every Day of Your Life!* Avon, Mass.: Adams Media, and F+W Publications Company, 2007.

Vernikos, Joan. *Sitting Kills, Moving Heals: How Everyday Movement Will Prevent Pain, Illness, and Early Death—and Exercise Alone Won't.* Fresno, Calif.: Quill Driver Books, 2011.

Websites

Introduction video to Tai Chi by Jet Li's Online Academy: https://www.youtube.com/watch?v=4VNw8tM7MYE

Tips and Strategies for Seniors: http://www.beginnerstaichi.com/learn-tai-chi-for-seniors.html

Warm Up Exercises for Tai Chi Workout: http://www.beginnerstaichi.com/tai-chi-exercises-for-beginners.html

20 Minute Home Yoga Workout for Beginners: https://www.youtube.com/watch?v=v7AYKMP6rOE

Featured Yoga Articles: http://www.yogabasics.com/

Yoga for Beginners by Yoga Journal: http://www.yogajournal.com/category/beginners/

Products

"Classical Stretch/Essentrics Workout" by Essentrics Online Streaming: http://classicalstretch.com/

Toning for Beginners DVD: http://www.essentrics.com/page/product-details/all/Toning_for_Beginners_DVD.htm

Endnotes, Chapter 4

1. Vernikos, Joan. *Sitting Kills, Moving Heals: How Everyday Movement Will Prevent Pain, Illness, and Early Death—and Exercise Alone Won't.* Fresno, Calif.: Quill Driver Books, 2011. 52.

2. Levine, James A. *Get Up!: Why Your Chair is Killing You and What You Can Do About It.* New York: St. Martin's Press LLC, 2014, 122-123.

3. Yang, Y, Verkuilen JV, Rosengren KS, Grubisich SA, Reed MR, and Hsiao-Wecksler ET. "Taijii and Qigong Training on Balance Mechanisms: A Randomized Controlled Trial of Older Adults." *Medical Science Monitor*, 2007: 339-348.

4. Zhang, J, K IshikawaTakata, H Yamazaki, T Morita, and T Ohta. "The Effects of Tai Chi Chuan on Physiological Function and Fear of Falling in the Less Robust Elderly: An Intervention Study for Preventing Falls." *Arch Grontol Geriatric*, 2006: 107-116.

5. Esmonde-White, Miranda. *Aging Backwards: Reverse the Aging Process and Look 10 Years Younger in 30 Minutes a Day.* New York: HarperCollins Books, 2014, 80.

CHAPTER 5

Eat What You Are Made Of...

What follows is the most in-depth chapter in the book, and for good reason. The truth that "your food is your medicine" has been known for centuries. Today, thousands of books and articles, hundreds of Internet sites, and scores of documentaries are devoted to this subject, and these information sources are growing daily. As more people are choosing natural alternatives to allopathic medicine and the market for organic food increases wildly, larger segments of the population are recognizing that health is intimately influenced by how the body is nourished, or not nourished. Like so many others who are approaching or experiencing elderhood, you probably want to know: What should I eat? What should I avoid eating? How can I maximize energy, strength and flexibility through my dietary choices? How can I support my life in the healthiest and most "youthing" fashion possible?

My overall answer to these questions is found in the title of this chapter: *Eat what you are made of...*! In the pages that follow, you will learn about the basic components of your "self"—what your body is composed of—and what factors truly nurture it, and what nutrients build your physical and total self.

As we explore the basic chemical and nutrient aspects of your body, I will be offering immediate practical suggestions for enhancing your diet, including some means of lifestyle adjustment to maximize these suggestions.

For those who would rather skip the rationale and jump immediately to the "Nutritional Bottom Line" (what to include and what to avoid) of diet and nutrition, look ahead to pages 97 and 101. These, at least, will be a highly useful guide for you. However, for maximum advantage, try to get the big picture. Understanding what you are made of will give you a framework on which to build a stronger, healthier body, and a more vibrant life.

OVERVIEW

Chemical elements, some of which are considered to be nutrient minerals, are the most basic building blocks of the earth itself and all its life forms. Various combinations of elements comprise the most familiar food categories: proteins, carbohydrates and fats. These three categories are considered to be **macronutrients**, meaning that they are large-molecule nutrients. To continue to have strong muscles, bones, skin, hair, teeth and organs, it is imperative to replenish your body with unadulterated, fresh sources of proteins, carbohydrates and fats frequently, preferably with each meal.

Your body's proteins, carbohydrates and fats begin to break down in short order and gradually become toxic residue rather than components of your strong body. If this biological waste is not efficiently processed, removed from your tissues and excreted, toxicity, inflammation and disease may ensue. Evidence of this type of macronutrient breakdown can be seen by looking in your compost container or garbage can.

Micronutrients are much smaller, yet vital substances. These include vitamins and the specific nutrient minerals (certain elements) that are required to sustain your body's critical functions, and life itself. Much of the vitamin content in your bodily tissues is water-soluble. Because these vitamins are flushed out of your system regularly, replenishment is necessary. The remaining vitamins are fat-soluble. They will reside in your body for several days before being degraded and eventually flushed down the toilet. Consistent and repetitive vitamin and mineral intake is critically important.

By itself, your body cannot manufacture these essential macro- and micronutrients, but instead requires proper feeding to resupply them and thus maintain optimal function. One challenge for many of us is that our culture lures us to make dietary choices based on taste and texture rather than on consideration of what nutrients our bodies need.

In this chapter you have the opportunity to learn about what your body *is made of*, which determines the nutrients and food sources it requires.

Let's take a closer look at the basic building blocks of your body, the elements.

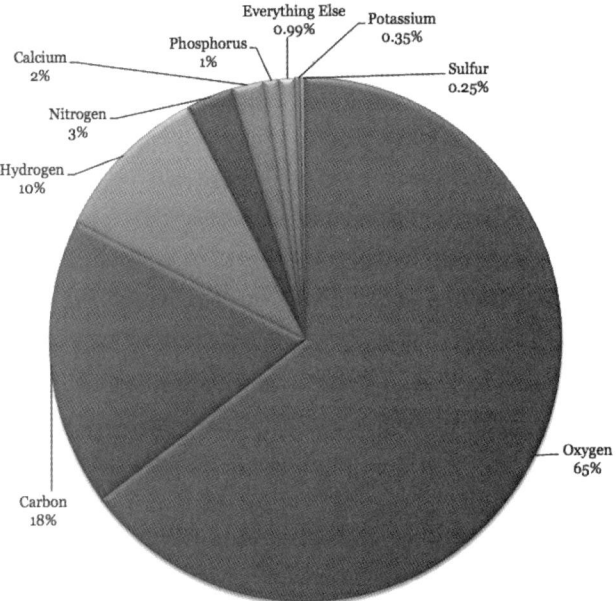

**Human Body Composition by Element
(Portioned by Mass Percent)**

Your Body's Elements

As you can see in the chart above, the six most prevalent elements in your body (oxygen, carbon, hydrogen, nitrogen, calcium, phosphorous) constitute approximately ninety-nine percent of its physical substance. Currently (2017), it is widely accepted that roughly two-thirds of the ninety (or ninety-two) naturally-occurring elements are required for the structures and functions of the human body. There are literally hundreds of thousands of necessary and complicated biological chemicals in your body, each composed of a unique **element** and **nutrient** formula. These elements do not function as independent elements, but synergistically operate in harmony with many other components in your body.

Eat What You Are Made Of... 55

> Carbon, hydrogen, nitrogen and oxygen are not considered to be nutrient minerals. They are essential **elements** in all living cells.

Oxygen

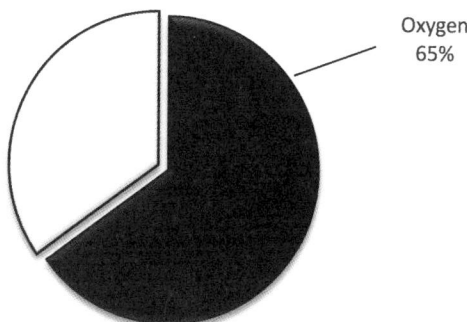

Oxygen
65%

Oxygen is the most prevalent element in your body and accounts for approximately sixty-five percent of your body weight. Typically, we think of oxygen as the life-giving component in the air we breathe. Relaxed but deep breathing is an excellent way to ramp up the fresh oxygen supply for your body. As you may recall from the previous chapter, *Pranayama* is the study and practice of purposeful deep breathing. It is a worthwhile undertaking. All of your life you have been routinely and unconsciously resupplying your body with oxygen. Often this has resulted in shallow breathing, which doesn't take full advantage of available oxygen. It makes sense to consciously practice deeper and more purposeful oxygen replenishment.

Since green plants release oxygen into their immediate environment, including them in your home or office may give you another slight oxygen edge. Walking or standing while consciously breathing in a forest or even in an enclosed botanical garden or greenhouse can also add a new dimension to your oxygen replacement efforts. Just for the fun of it, consider visiting an oxygen bar (found in many cities, airports and shopping malls) to receive a thirty-minute "shot" of "high-octane" oxygen that is often administered with your choice of healthful essential oils.

Water intake is another major source of oxygen because each water molecule is composed of two hydrogen atoms and one oxygen atom. Drinking pure water may provide more health benefits than you may have expected (see section on Water later in this chapter). Including fresh and raw fruits and vegetables in your diet will also provide some water and even oxygen.

Oxygen is also a component in each of the three macronutrients: **proteins, carbohydrates and fats**. Foods that promote your red blood cell supply can be considered helpful in your overall oxygen utilization. Proteins from animal and plant sources, especially those that contain iron, help your body build healthy red blood cells. This creates higher levels of hemoglobin (the oxygen-carrying molecule in your red blood cells) that assist in the transport and utilization of the oxygen you breathe.

If you know or suspect that you have an oxygen deficiency, you need to be working with your healthcare practitioner and using medical oxygen at their specifically prescribed dose. In addition, you can consider the above recommendations and consult your natural healthcare practitioner for specific nutritional recommendations that, over time, have the potential to improve your body's oxygen saturation. I have successfully helped several patients with specific homeopathic remedies that allowed them to tolerate traveling and hiking at higher elevations (in some cases by 2000 to 3000 feet) after treatment and supplementation.

> Oxygen deficiency is qualified by a reading on your pulse oximeter below 90 percent oxygen saturation. You should check in with your healthcare provider, as each case may vary.

Carbon

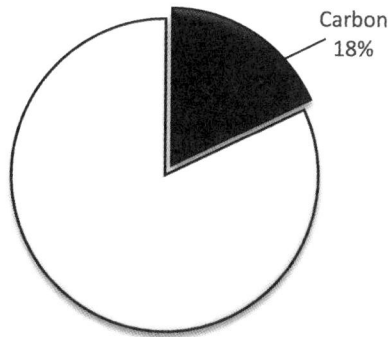

Carbon is found in all living organisms and comprises approximately eighteen percent of your body's weight. It is the primary structural component in carbohydrate molecules. The word "carbohydrate" derives from the biochemical process that forms it—hydration of carbon. During photosynthesis, plants make carbohydrates by combining carbon and water (hydrogen and oxygen). Carbon is also present in proteins and fats. Every known vitamin contains a carbon-based "backbone."

Carbon is a structural component of every biological molecule, cell, tissue and organism. Its presence distinguishes living matter (organic matter) from non-living (inorganic matter). We encounter this interesting substance as a solid that manifests outside of our bodies as coal, graphite and diamonds. In its gaseous form, carbon dioxide feeds forests, crops and gardens.

> Activated charcoal capsules and powder are wonderful detoxifiers because carbon is a highly reactive element that perpetually wants to combine with others. It effortlessly attaches to and neutralizes offending toxins. You can also clean stubborn stains off your teeth by brushing them with activated charcoal, but it can be a bit messy.

Nuts, fruits and vegetables are rich sources of carbon. Avocados and olives are two of the highest sources. Because carbon is readily available and easily incorporated into your body, it is not an element that you need to search out or supplement. By following the general principle of **eating what you are made of**, you will undoubtedly consume adequate quantities of carbon that your body can incorporate into the structural building blocks—proteins, carbohydrates and fats—in order to build your connective tissues, including teeth, hair, skin and nails.

Hydrogen

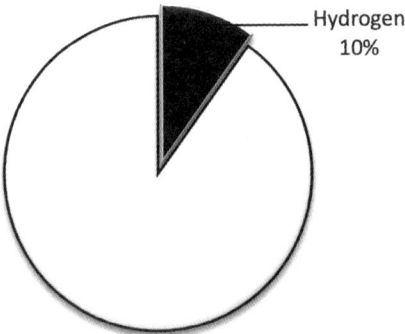

Hydrogen is the lightest-weight element of all and also happens to be the most common element in the universe. Because it is so light, it is not predominant in the earth's atmosphere. (It is believed that much of the free hydrogen left the earth's atmosphere and rose high up into outer space. Many stars, planets and novas are largely composed of hydrogen, including our sun.) Your body contains more hydrogen atoms than any other type. Due to its light nature, hydrogen only accounts for ten percent of your body's total weight.

We encounter hydrogen primarily in the form of water; two thirds of all water is hydrogen. Two hydrogen atoms plus one oxygen atom form a molecule of water. In Greek, the root words of hydrogen mean "water forming." Biologically active chemicals include proteins, amino acids, carbohydrates, fats, vitamins, enzymes and hormones. They are often termed "biochemicals." Hydrogen is a component of each of these categories of biochemicals.

Your stomach's hydrochloric acid is derived from hydrogen and triggers your body's production of digestive enzymes. These enzymes help to break down and repurpose proteins. Hydrogen is also used by your body as a buffering agent to help regulate its inherent acid/alkaline balance. The process for measuring acidity versus alkalinity in the body is called pH testing. This chemical symbol stands for either potential of hydrogen or power of hydrogen.

> **Testing Your pH**
> Litmus paper (or more specific pH test paper) can be used to assess the acid/alkaline balance of bodily fluids, most often urine and/or saliva. You can get this test paper at local healthfood store, online, or through your healthcare practitioner.
>
> Numerous health and metabolic conditions can affect your pH reading. If you test your first urine of the day, I find that a pH reading between 7.4 and 7.6 is optimal. If your reading is in the 5 or 6 range, you do not have enough hydrogen (a component of bicarbonate) circulating to properly buffer the biological acids that your body produces.
>
> To take a reading, simply dip your test paper into your fresh urine sample. Compare the color of your test strip to the chart on its container. Record the date and time of your test next to your test results. Test and record at least once daily in the morning before eating for one week. The average of these seven tests is your baseline pH. If your average is below 7.4, continue to test daily while adding alkalizing foods and/or beverages as discussed in the following box.

Before you test alkalinizing foods or beverages with Clinical Kinesiology you should refer to page xvii in the Introduction to refresh yourself on the appropriate steps and methods for this testing.

Your dietary sources for hydrogen are abundant: water, fats, carbohydrates and proteins. Especially noteworthy hydrogen foods include cabbage, carrots, celery, legumes, meats, spinach, watermelon and tomatoes.

From Acid to Alkaline
The addition of alkalinizing foods or beverages to your diet, based on your daily testing of the body's pH level can be beneficial. Some healthy and alkalinizing foods include grapefruit*, lemon juice and water, asparagus, and commercially prepared kombucha tea. You may also consider modifying your diet to include mostly fresh vegetables for several days in order to optimize your pH reading by bringing it closer to 7.4 or above. I encourage you to use Clinical Kinesiology testing to select among the proposed food and beverage choices.

* Remember that **grapefruit juice** is contraindicated for many pharmaceutical medications. You will have to specifically check with your pharmacist or prescribing physician about eating whole **grapefruit** in combination with any medication in question.

Warning about Hydrogen…
You should **avoid foods labeled "hydrogenated" or "partially hydrogenated."** These are usually vegetable oils or shortenings that have been chemically and thermally altered and forced to absorb extra hydrogen to provide increased shelf life for the product. This dramatically alters the product. Your body cannot properly process it. The hydrogenation process is incompatible with human longevity.

Nitrogen

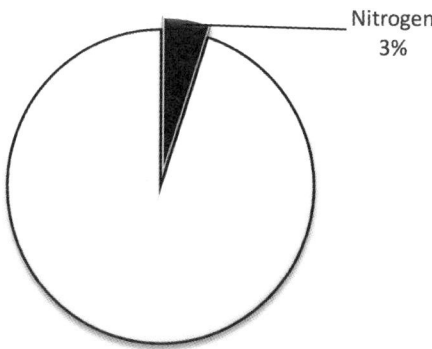

Although nitrogen constitutes only three percent of your body, it fills over seventy-eight percent of the earth's atmosphere. Nitrogen gas (N_2, indicating two nitrogen atoms closely bound together) is floating all around you, but it is totally unusable by your body in this form. Each dyad of nitrogen atoms must be reconfigured to become usable by living beings. Breathing in nitrogen from the air provides no benefit.

Luckily for us, nature has provided at least two viable ways to make nitrogen available to biological systems. The first method is rather dramatic: each lightning strike provides the energy to reconfigure water and nitrogen gas to form naturally occurring nitrates and ammonia, which fall as rain and soak into the soil providing nourishment for plants.

The second method is accomplished by the action of beneficial bacteria and algae found in healthy soil. The earth's microbiome (community of probiotic microorganisms in the soil) is composed of colonies of soil-based bacteria. These function similarly to the friendly intestinal bacteria in your body, which contribute to overall human health. These soil bacteria "fix" the nitrogen for its use by tiny plant rootlets. The result is more robust and nutritious plant life. When we consume fruits and vegetables, we consume useable nitrogen.

Nitrogen is critically important to your body because it is present in every single amino acid, and therefore every single protein molecule in your structure. Nitrogen is required for your DNA and your RNA as well. In other words, your very life depends on usable nitrogen coming into your body regularly. If your water supply is well water or spring water, you may gain a minor amount of usable nitrogen from this source.

The best way to procure usable nitrogen for your body is to eat a variety of fresh fruits and vegetables that have been grown with care. If you or your local farmer's market vendors follow a chemical-free and soil-enriching philosophy in growing produce, the usable nitrogen level in those plants will be maximized. Adding compostable biomass—including scraps of vegetable matter, leaves, twigs, straw, ashes from your fireplace or campfire, and even weeds that you have pulled (but discarded the seed heads from)—is a simple and earth-friendly way to provide more nitrogen to the soil.

> **Homemade, Natural, Nitrogen-Rich Fertilizer**
> "Compost tea"—made from the herbs stinging nettles and or comfrey—is a powerful and inexpensive nitrogen booster for your garden, whether you grow in small containers or use an entire garden plot. Compost tea is a wonderful enrichment for any garden, but most needed when plants are abnormally pale or yellow. Both comfrey and stinging nettles are hardy perennials in most moderate climates.
>
> To make compost tea, start with a suitable container such as a two- or five-gallon bucket. Fill the bottom third with coarsely chopped or torn comfrey or stinging nettles leaves (be sure to wear substantial gloves and long sleeves), and then fill with water to about three inches below the rim of your container. Cover the container to prevent evaporation, but leave it in a warm and sunny place if possible. The sunlight will heat and brew your compost tea within two to six weeks. Then you can strain the solids (use this as mulch around the base of your plants or add to the compost pile) and apply the liquid to your plants. You can also consider your compost tea to be a concentrate and add portions to your watering can at intervals.

Especially nitrogen-rich vegetables are asparagus, beets, broccoli, Brussels sprouts, chestnuts, lettuce, radishes, rhubarb and spinach. Most animal foods (meat, dairy, eggs, fish and poultry) are high in protein and therefore high in nitrogen as well. Remember to select the most naturally grown and produced items—organic and chemical-free when possible.

> **Avoid the Artificials**
> Recognize that artificially added nitrates, nitrites or nitrosamines do not efficiently yield usable nitrogen and present numerous health risks, so avoid them. High-temperature cooking or frying of meats preserved with nitrites can convert the preservative to the more problematic chemical nitrosamine. These chemicals function as preservatives and are often found in cured or processed meats and meat products, processed cheese foods, some beers and some cosmetics, and are closely linked to several kinds of cancers.

> **About L-argentine**
> Use of the precursor nutrient, L-arginine, is gaining status in the nutritional world as a promoter of cardiovascular health. This benefit is due to your body's ability to transform it into nitric oxide. After swallowing a capsule or powdered source, the amino acid L-arginine releases its nitrogen into your system and both soothes and heals the inner linings of your blood vessels, ultimately providing increased blood flow.

These four major elements—oxygen, carbon, hydrogen, nitrogen—are similar in the respect that they are prevalent in our environment. They are not considered to be minerals, and we are not typically deficient in any one of these "Big Four Elements." However, this is not the case with other elements, the **nutrient minerals.** Deficiencies in this area are common, and precipitate serious health consequences.

ESSENTIAL NUTRIENTS OVERVIEW

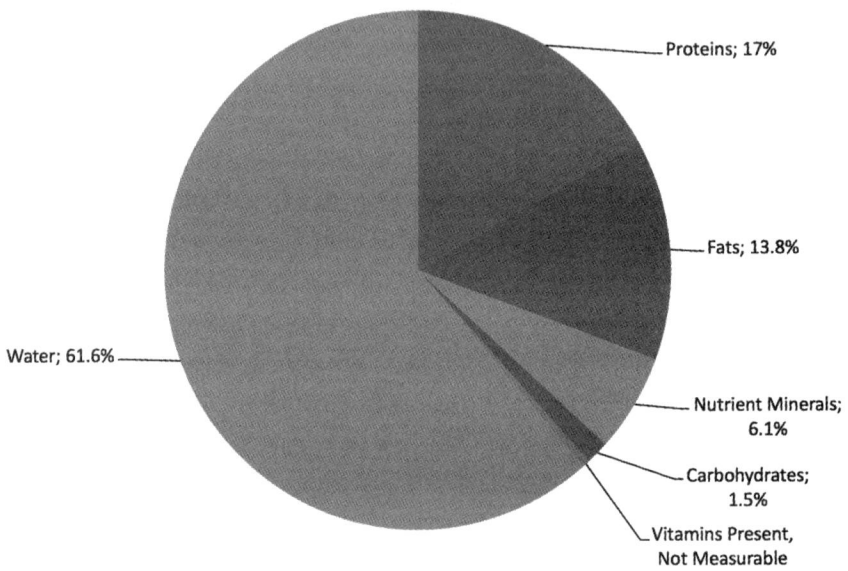

Human Body Composition by Essential Nutrient Categories (Portioned by Mass Percent)

- Proteins; 17%
- Fats; 13.8%
- Nutrient Minerals; 6.1%
- Carbohydrates; 1.5%
- Vitamins Present, Not Measurable
- Water; 61.6%

Essential nutrients must be consistently supplied to your body. They participate in the construction of cells, tissues, organs and all body structures. These essential nutrients participate in all natural biochemical reactions, and must be supplied by your dietary and water intake, and for many of us with supplemental nutrients.

YOUR BODY'S MICRONUTRIENTS

The first category of essential nutrients is called micronutrients and includes **nutrient minerals** and **vitamins.** Nutrient minerals (elements) are used to construct all the other essential nutrients. Vitamins are built of various elements and other biological compounds called amino acids. Vitamins help your body perform biochemical functions and serve as chemical catalysts for metabolism, digestion, absorption, and other countless miracles that take place in your body.

Nutrient Minerals

This category of elements that compose our bodies is characteristically different from the "Big Four" (oxygen, carbon, nitrogen and hydrogen). **Nutrient minerals, or dietary minerals**, which include calcium, phosphorus, potassium, sulfur, and many more, must be consumed daily (or at least frequently). Refer back to "The Human Body Composition by Element" chart on page 54.

A wise form of "nutrient insurance" is to take a comprehensive multi-mineral supplement on a regular basis. Including these supplements in your daily routine will improve your cellular and organ function, and strengthen your hair, skin, teeth and nails.

Many good nutrient-mineral formulations exist. One of my favorites is T. J. Clark's Legendary Colloidal Mineral Formula™. This is a liquid formula that I add to my morning water with fresh squeezed lemon juice, daily. When choosing a mineral formula you can certainly utilize your Clinical Kinesiology skills to test a variety of formulations for compatibility with your body.

Professional Testing with Clinical Kinesiology

Individuals who are debilitated, have chronic or dramatic health issues, or pronounced deficiencies of specific minerals should be tested by a professional Clinical Kinesiologist. An experienced Clinical Kinesiologist should be able to test specific mineral needs and design an appropriate program for an individual. Specific handmodes have been discovered for testing most of the nutrient minerals.

> **Nutrient Minerals**
>
> **Elements:** Each mineral is a specific element. Approximately forty elements are currently understood to participate in the structure of the human body. It is not yet been determined whether all of these are considered to be essential micronutrients.
>
> **Approximate percentage of body weight:** 6.1 percent
>
> **Biological Purpose:** Necessary for both biochemical enzyme and digestive enzyme function; serve to conduct nerve impulses (body electricity) that is needed to transport messages through your nerves to all body parts, including all muscles, even your heart; provide the framework of the entire body's structure; actively participate in transferring nutrients into your cells.
>
> **Biochemical Classification:** Inorganic
>
> **Food energy potential:** 0 Calories/gram, not a source of food energy.
>
> **Required enzymes:** Unspecified: The food substrates containing the minerals must be well digested so that the body can absorb the mineral.

Calcium

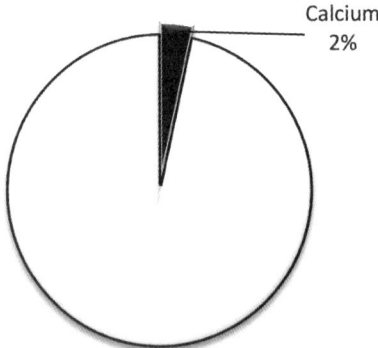

The most prevalent nutrient mineral in your body is calcium. It comprises two percent of your body's structure. Calcium's most common job is to build and maintain the structural integrity of your skeleton and teeth.

Ninety-nine percent of your body's stored calcium is found in your bony structures, while the other one percent is necessary for nerve and muscle function and complex biochemical and enzymatic processes.

As we age, our ability to absorb and utilize calcium diminishes. For some people, this diminishment is quite dramatic. When a person's total absorbed calcium falls short of their required amount, significant changes happen. A person's wise body "steals" the necessary calcium from the bone structure and diverts it to life-sustaining enzymatic and biochemical processes. If this "calcium-deficit spending" pattern persists, bone loss occurs and progresses to osteoporosis.

Some of the calcium-dependent biochemical processes that our bodies perform on a daily basis are considered bio-electrical tasks.

> **Bio-electrical Functions That Require Calcium (also magnesium, potassium and several trace minerals)**
> - Heart rhythm regulation
> - Balanced muscle contractility
> - Blood pressure regulation
> - Balanced nerve function
> - Proper nerve conduction
> - Balanced thought processing and brain wave production
> - Sleep cycle regulation

When calcium is not effectively absorbed and/or utilized or not proportionally balanced with other nutrient minerals—such as magnesium, potassium, phosphorus and numerous trace minerals—a broad variety of maladies may develop.

> **Symptoms of Calcium Deficiency or Dysfunction**
> - Colon polyps and colon cancer
> - Depression
> - Heart rate irregularities   *(continued on next page)*

- High blood pressure
- High cholesterol
- Impaired kidney function
- Impaired wound healing and scab formation
- Impairment of necessary blood clotting
- Inefficient heart contractions
- Insomnia
- Muscle cramping and spasms
- Obesity or difficult weight control
- Preeclampsia
- Various hormonal imbalances
- Weakening of bones: osteopenia, osteoporosis, fractures
- Weakening of teeth: cavities, cracked or broken teeth

Do My Bones Need More Than Calcium?

Calcium combined with magnesium and phosphorus is similar to a honeycomb structure and gives shape and strength to your bones. These three nutrient minerals are the most prevalent, but not the only important components of your strong bones. In this analogy the "honey" within the hexagonal spaces consists of the synergistic nutrient components that are absolutely necessary for bone integrity.

WHAT ARE MY BONES MADE OF?

Minerals	Vitamins	Amino Acids	Macronutrients
Boron	Vitamin C	L-lysine	Protein
Calcium	Vitamin D	Proline	
Copper	Vitamin K		
Magnesium			
Manganese			
Phosphorus			
Silica			
Various trace minerals			
Zinc			

Traces of other important nutrients are likely required for healthy bones and will be identified by researchers and scientists in the future. This honeycomb example clearly illustrates how synergistic and dynamically interactive the elements, nutrient minerals, vitamins, amino acids, proteins, carbohydrates and fats are in your body. We can consider that these same nutritional components are necessary in varying proportions for all of your body's tissues. The most important principle to remember is that the above synergistic formula, which includes each of these critical body-building and body-supporting nutrients, must be present with no significant alterations for optimal strength and health. When your skin, hair and fingernails are robust and firm, it is likely that your bones are as well.

A Diverse Selection of Calcium-Rich Foods

Mother Nature plans quite well. She provides absorbable calcium in numerous tasty food sources. The first category people generally think of when it comes to calcium is dairy. It is important to remember to choose dairy products with no added hormones, especially the synthetic growth hormones used for cattle. When selecting dairy products, opt for pasture-raised and organic versions, and for whole milk rather than lo-fat or processed varieties. Raw milk, provided by conscientious dairies, is most preferable. Pasture-raised cattle produce richer milk. This milk is particularly rich in vitamin K, which helps your calcium utilization. Properly handled raw milk has a higher amount of vitamins (C, B_6, B_{12}), probiotics, intact enzymes and proteins than pasteurized milk.

Sources for Safe Raw Milk and Organic Pasture Fed Dairy Items
- Local organic farms and dairies
- Farmer's markets
- Buy a share of a cow or goat
- Consult Farm to Consumer Legal Defense Fund (www.farmtoconsumer.org/) and Campaign for Real Milk (www.realmilk.com)

> **Bovine Hormones**
> Recombinant Bovine Somatotropin (rBST) and Recombinant Bovine Growth Hormone (rbGH) are growth hormones commonly used in dairy farming. These do not provide benefits to humans and may interfere with your hormone balance.

Another important criterion is to seek out GMO-free dairy products, meaning that the cows or goats were not fed genetically modified feed.

> **GMOs**
> Genetically altered food items and those **not certified** GMO-free are closely correlated with various disease processes, leaky gut syndrome, gastrointestinal disturbances, and even a variety of cancers.[1]

Other categories of calcium-rich foods include seeds, nuts, fruits and vegetables. By adhering to the dietary principles above and consistently eating a rotating selection of foods from the following list, you will supply calcium to your body regularly.

Dairy Products	Nuts and Seeds	Vegetables	Fruits
Buttermilk	Almonds	Bok choy	Figs
Cheddar cheese	Pistachio nuts	Broccoli	Papaya
Swiss cheese	Quinoa	Brussels sprouts	
Whole milk	Sesame seeds	Dried beans (black, black-eyed peas, garbanzo, pinto, edamame)	
Whole milk kefir		Globe artichokes	
Whole milk yogurt		Kale	
		Peas	
		Rutabaga	

The addition of a balanced, supplemental nutrient-mineral formula is a proactive step for most of us to consider as we age. Many calcium formulations are available and choosing one that is right for you and your situation takes careful consideration.

> **Calcium Choices: Less or More**
>
> Calcium carbonate is the least expensive form of calcium, and in my opinion is the least beneficial. Often this form is sourced from ground oyster shells or chalky mineral deposits. Anyone with sub-optimal digestive function will be more challenged to make use of this form. Common antacid tablets, such as Tums®, are also generally ineffective since they are designed to limit the available acidity in your stomach, and therefore will diminish mineral absorption from food or supplements.
>
> A concentrated food-source supplement of calcium and other minerals is likely to be the best absorbed. Consult your natural healthcare practitioner.

Colloidal calcium or calcium citrate in a liquid mineral formula is generally well absorbed by most people. Calcium lactate, calcium glycinate, calcium malate and calcium orotate are other absorbable forms. For many people the wisest choice will be to have the guidance of a nutritionist, a Clinical Kinesiologist or your trusted natural healthcare provider initially. Once you are pointed in the right direction by an expert, you may choose to compare various calcium and/or mineral combinations using your Clinical Kinesiology skills to find which formula tests the strongest for your body. Periodically rotate or change your mineral formula. Refresh yourself in the principles of proper muscle testing by referring to page xvii in the introduction of this book.

> **The Acid Environment**
> Calcium (as well as many other important minerals) is best absorbed in an acidic environment. Maintaining proper acidity in your stomach will help you absorb calcium from foods and supplemental nutrients. Drinking water with lemon juice or apple cider vinegar prior to ingesting meals and supplements is one simple method. Taking a hydrochloric acid digestive aid is another. ***Remember to brush your teeth after consuming lemon juice or apple cider vinegar to protect your tooth enamel.

Lifestyle Factors That Can Diminish Your Calcium Absorption
Many lifestyle factors can diminish individual components required for bone and tissue integrity, skewing the recipe and weakening your body's structure. Minimal coffee and alcohol consumption may not produce a significant reduction of calcium and its friends in your body; however, excessive or daily use of these solvents *will* flush calcium and many other nutrient minerals and vitamins from your system. Smoking is shown to reduce levels of vitamin A, most B vitamins, vitamin C, selenium and zinc as well as the amino acid cysteine, and is known to promote osteoporosis.[2] Research has definitively shown that smoking

> **Medications That Interfere with Calcium Absorption and Utilization**[3]
> - Acid blockers
> - Antacids
> - Antibiotics
> - Aspirin and aspirin compounds
> - Blood pressure medication
> - Heart medications (Digoxin and calcium channel blockers)
> - Steroids (oral or inhaled)
> - Synthetic hormones
> - Thyroid medications

and tobacco use directly inhibit your body's ability to both absorb calcium and to metabolize the calcium that was successfully absorbed. A variety of medications can also block calcium absorption in your body or even flush it from your system.

Phosphorus

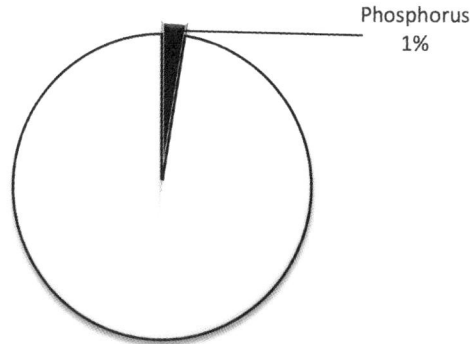

Phosphorus is a basic requirement for life, as it is present in every living cell. Phosphorus accounts for one percent of your body's weight, making it the fifth most prevalent element and the second most prevalent nutrient mineral in the human body. In your bones, calcium phosphate (hydroxyapatite) builds the honeycomb-like framework that gives strength to your teeth and bones, and allows "spaces" for other reinforcing trace minerals to nest.

In all living cells, phosphorus is compounded with other elements and important biological substances. In your body, biological phosphate (phosphorus bound to an oxygen molecule) is able to produce energy in the mitochondria (small "power plants") of your cells.

> **Phospholipids**
> All cell membranes are composed of phospholipids (phosphate linked to good fats, often cholesterol). Due to this flexible cell membrane structure, movement of body fluids and nutrients are specifically measured and regulated to allow the correct amounts of needed substances into and out of your cells.

Phosphorus is responsible, at least in part, for the function of numerous enzymes and hormones, movement of oxygen into living cells, production and replication of DNA and RNA and other energy producing chemical reactions. In addition, compounded phosphorus helps hydrogen regulate your acid-base balance, or pH. In short, phosphorus plays a part in almost every biological and cellular job performed inside your body.

Eat Your Phosphorus

Essentially, all foods contain some usable phosphorus compounds in the form of bioavailable phosphates. Therefore, true phosphorus deficiency is rarely seen, except in cases of starvation, premature birth or metabolic upheaval including some serious kidney disorders that may impair normal absorption of phosphorus. In other cases, individuals experiencing or recovering from diabetic ketoacidosis, alcoholism or serious respiratory compromise may also be deficient in phosphorus.

Prominent sources of phosphorus include salmon and other fish, turkey and chicken, dairy, eggs, grains, and nuts and seeds. Some nuts and grains are a bit difficult to digest since humans do not have the specific enzyme that would release phosphorus from the compound native to these concentrated foods. That being said, the human digestive tract is still able to process and utilize about one half of the phosphorus content in these foods. Soaking or sprouting (soak or sprout for twelve to thirty-six hours depending on the item) grains, nuts and seeds can further overcome the bioavailability obstacle.

Phosphorus is germane to all plants, so it is available in fruits and vegetables but less concentrated than is found in the proportionally higher protein foods. Selecting foods that were naturally grown with care also assures a higher natural phosphate content in your diet. Chemical-free growing methods and natural soil amendments in your personal garden or that of your chosen grower will yield more phosphorus in any crop.

Enhancing the Soil

Phosphorus deficient soil may require some detective work to identify. However, there are some obvious signs such as increased occurrence of disease, and delay in crop maturity and yield. Soils with deficiencies also produce plants with smaller-sized leaves, smaller seeds, fewer seeds and a diminished germination rate. The leaves of corn and tomatoes that are lacking sufficient phosphorus may develop an abnormal purple color.

Guano (manure from birds and bats) is a rich source of phosphorus for your garden. Zoos often sell bags of guano to gardeners. Adding compostable kitchen and garden waste will also increase the phosphorus and trace mineral content of your soil. Rotating the crops in your garden and working the dead foliage into the soil are other simple ways to promote consistent phosphorus in the soil content. Corn, soybeans and alfalfa are crops that pull greater amounts of phosphorus from the soil.

Lifestyle Factors That Contribute to Unbalanced Phosphorus

Drinking coffee and caffeine-containing tea are two lifestyle factors that can leach phosphorus and other minerals from your system

The amount of phosphorus in our bodies must be balanced with calcium, magnesium, vitamin D and many trace minerals. The phosphoric acid added to colas is responsible for skewing the proper mineral balance for many individuals. In effect, this excess phosphorus causes the body to eliminate calcium and slow the production of vitamin D resulting in osteoporosis for many unsuspecting soda drinkers. As some current research states, "Phosphorus intake in excess of the nutrient needs of healthy adults is thought to disrupt hormonal regulation of phosphorus (P), calcium (Ca), and vitamin D, contributing to impaired peak bone mass, bone reabsorption, and greater risk of fracture.[4]"

Medications That May Deplete Phosphorus[5]
- Acid-reducing medications
- Blood pressure medications
- Diuretics
- Estrogen and estrogen-containing drugs
- Laxatives

Potassium

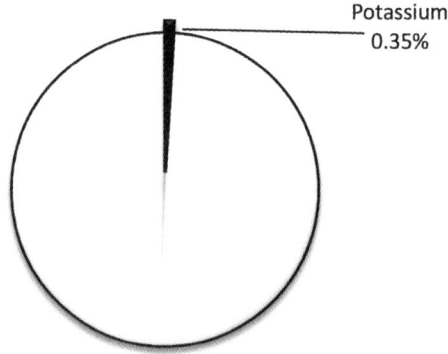

Potassium accounts for 0.35 percent of your body's composition. While potassium is most commonly found in your cells, it works in conjunction with sodium, which is most often found outside of your cells. The majority of this interaction occurs within your muscles, but it also occurs in your body's tissues to a much lesser degree. Your body exquisitely choreographs movement of these electrolyte nutrient minerals to exchange their positions relevant to the delicate cell membrane. This "dance" causes muscle contractions (and subsequent relaxations) for all of your muscle movements. This sodium-potassium pumping mechanism also provides the propulsion of nerve impulses down the length of any nerve that needs to convey a message to another part of your body.

Potassium helps stabilize the acid and alkaline balance in your body. This very important function directly affects many metabolic processes including assisting your body to metabolize other macro- and micronutrients. Potassium also plays a critical role in your body's necessary blood clotting process.

> **Potassium's Functions in Your Body**
> - Activates enzymes for metabolism
> - Attracts oxygen to the tissues
> - Balances and buffers body fluids
> - Promotes normal muscle contraction
> - Promotes normal nerve conductivity
> - Promotes immunity
> - Regulates balanced heart rhythm

"… Researchers concluded that higher potassium intake may protect postmenopausal women against ischemic stroke, death from all causes, and small vessel disease, especially if they do not have high blood pressure."[6] This article also indicates that the average intake of potassium by Americans is considerably lower than the amount needed to reduce the risk of stroke.

Too Much Potassium?

Excess potassium is problematic and can lead to death from cardiac arrest. Several health conditions and types of trauma may cause potassium to leak out of the cells into the bloodstream, raising the level dangerously. Chronic kidney disease, certain hormonal imbalances, and uncontrolled diabetes are a few examples of conditions that account for a majority of the cases involving critically elevated potassium. Rhabdomyolysis, commonly known as muscle degeneration, can be caused by severe trauma or serious burns. It may also be a dramatic side effect of statins and other prescription drugs. This condition causes potassium to leak into the blood stream and destroy muscle cells. In extreme cases, kidney damage and even death may occur. ACE inhibitors, or beta-blocker medications commonly prescribed for hypertension (high blood pressure), may also increase levels of potassium in the blood. Surgery may temporarily increase potassium levels during the tissue healing process. In addition, drug and/or alcohol abuse may cause elevated potassium levels as well as many other devastating health risks.

Excess potassium levels need to be closely monitored by electrolyte blood tests and evaluated by your doctor or healthcare practitioner. Common symptoms of excess potassium include a slower than normal heart rate, weak pulse, weak muscles, impaired mobility, difficulty with breathing, nausea, fatigue and tiredness. These symptoms are not conclusive and may occur for a variety of reasons. It is of utmost importance to have your blood tested if you have any inkling that your potassium level is out of balance.

Potassium Deficiency

Potassium within your body must be properly balanced with sodium, calcium, magnesium, iron, zinc, vitamin D and certain B vitamins or it will be excessively excreted from your body.

Potassium Deficiency Symptoms
- Abdominal bloating
- Cardiovascular symptoms ranging from angina and heart rhythm irregularity to stroke
- Colitis
- Diarrhea
- Diminished kidney and/or adrenal function
- Diminished reflexes
- Dry skin or acne
- Emotional detachment and mental confusion
- Glucose intolerance
- Infertility
- Insomnia
- Irregular breathing and/or shortness of breath
- Muscular weakness even developing into intermittent paralysis
- Slow growth in infants and children

Potassium deficiency can be triggered by chronic diarrhea and/or vomiting. You may also lose potassium through your sweat. In all of these scenarios, hydrating with water or an appropriate electrolyte fluid can quickly reestablish your fluids and electrolytes, including potassium.

Diabetic ketoacidosis, a serious condition in which your blood becomes too acidic from lack of insulin or blood sugar control, can cause your body to excrete potassium excessively. Kidney disease also affects potassium levels and may either cause your body to excessively excrete or retain potassium. Certain eating disorders may result in potassium deficiency as well.

> **Recipe for a Homemade Electrolyte Replacement Drink**
> Stir together:
> 1 quart of pure water
> 1/2 teaspoon of sea salt or Real Salt®
> 1/2 teaspoon of baking soda
> OPTIONAL: 1/2 cup of freshly squeezed fruit juice for flavor

In the event that you cannot appropriately rehydrate yourself due to prolonged vomiting or diarrhea, you will need to visit the emergency room for intravenous rehydration. Potassium chloride (KCl) probably will be added to your saline IV. Proper administration of this potassium is critical. Adding potassium directly to your bloodstream too rapidly may cause serious heart rhythm abnormalities and even death. That is why your nurse should be checking your IV frequently. Abnormalities demonstrated on an electrocardiogram in a dehydrated person with diminished potassium can be shown to normalize in a short time after receiving an appropriate dosage of potassium chloride intravenously.

Potassium is easily accessed by eating many natural, healthful foods.

| Potassium Foods |||
Fruit	Vegetables	Other
Apricots	Beet greens	Clams
Avocados	Bok choy	Halibut
Bananas	Broccoli	Mackerel
Beets	Brussels sprouts	Red snapper
Grapefruit	Cabbage	Yogurt
Honeydew melon	Cauliflower	
Oranges	Collard greens	
Prunes and prune juice	Dried beans, especially adzuki, kidney, Lima and white beans	
Tomatoes and tomato juice	Mushrooms	

Lifestyle Factors That Diminish Potassium

High endurance or heavy exercise that induces profuse sweating, or excessive time in the sauna without rehydrating and replacing balanced electrolytes, can precipitate a potassium deficiency. Excess sodium intake (typically from table salt, sodium chloride, rather than a balanced mineral salt) can also push potassium out of your body leading to a deficiency. Consuming caffeinated beverages, including coffee, tea and soda, can potentially disrupt your potassium levels. People with chronic headaches, diabetes or hypoglycemia may also have a slight potassium deficiency.

Medications That Diminish Potassium[7]
- Acid blockers and antacids
- Antibiotics
- Anticonvulsants
- Blood pressure medications
- Bronchodilators
- Laxatives and stool softeners
- Parkinson's medications
- Steroids and other hormones

Sulfur

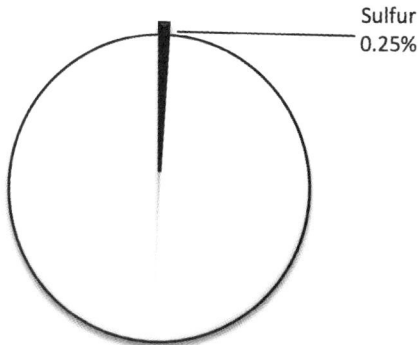

Sulfur has a fairly unusual personality and it's worth mentioning a few of its quirks. Some sulfur deposits rode into earth's atmosphere on meteorites and crashed into the rocky crust of the planet long ago. This celestial sulfur smashed into the mix of elements present at its landing site. Even today, volcanic eruptions spew sulfur skyward; then it ultimately falls back to earth. One quarter of one percent, 0.25 percent, of your body is composed of sulfur.

Sulfur delights in stimulating your senses. Pure sulfur is bright yellow and totally odorless, while sulfur-containing compounds (naturally occurring sulfates and sulfites) release the sulfur odor. Sometimes it distinctly resembles rotten eggs. Other times it has the fragrance of broccoli or the odor of your urine shortly after eating asparagus. The health benefits of the strong-smelling vegetables—onions and garlic—are partially due to the sulfur they contain. Skunks also utilize a sulfur compound when they spray a plume of their characteristic fragrance.

While you are relaxing and soaking in your favorite hot springs you may immediately smell a sulfate fragrance. A bit later you may notice the skin-soothing and smoothing effect of sulfur from the warm and tranquilizing water.

> ### A Sulfur Bath
> Epsom salt is magnesium sulfate, adding one to two cups of these granules to your warm bathwater allows your skin to absorb both of these useful elements.

Sulfur in Your Body

This feisty yellow nutrient mineral contributes to forming many cellular and tissue structures including your hair, skin, teeth, muscles, bones and connective tissues. The bile produced in your liver to digest fatty foods contains high amounts of sulfur. Sulfur-containing amino acids assist your liver to detoxify various toxins and even toxic metals from your body.

Sulforaphane-containing cruciferous vegetables are known to deter many types of cancer.[8] More recent research indicates that sulforaphane has neuro-protective effects for people who have had traumatic spinal cord injury, or neuro-degenerative problems such as Alzheimer's disease and Parkinson's disease.[9]

Sulfur-Containing Compounds in Your Body		
Amino Acids	**Vitamins**	**Tissue compounds**
Cysteine	Biotin (B_7)	Chondroitin sulfate (in joints)
Glutathione	Thiamine (B_1)	Collagen (in skin and muscles)
Methionine		Keratin (in hair and nails)
Taurine		Tissue proteins

Sulfur Deficiency

Sulfur deficiency is rare, but can occur in cases of starvation and extremely low protein diets. Mild sulfur deficiency may occur if a person's normal intestinal microbiome (necessary helpful bacteria) is damaged; their ability to break down and utilize sulfur compounds may be negatively impacted. Sub-optimal sulfur levels may occur if foods are grown in sulfur-depleted soil. Hair breakage and loss are clues to sulfur deficiency. Skin rashes and lesions are other indicators.

Sulfur in Your Food

Sulfur is commonly found in the cruciferous vegetable family including broccoli, cauliflower, cabbage and kale. The flowers of these vegetables are often yellow, signaling the presence of sulfur. (You can consider eating the flowers and sprouts of your cruciferous vegetables as an additional healthy food option.) Sulfur is also found in the allium family that includes onions, garlic, leaks and chives. Other rich sulfur food sources include high protein food choices from both the plant and animal kingdoms.

Sulfur-Containing Foods
- Arugula*
- Asparagus
- Bananas
- Bok choy*
- Broccoli (all forms)*
- Brussels sprouts*
- Cabbage*
- Cauliflower*
- Collard greens*
- Dairy products
- Dandelions
- Eggs
- Garlic
- Grapefruit
- Kale*
- Lemon
- Meats
- Mustard greens and seeds*
- Onions
- Pineapple
- Radishes(all types)*
- Rutabaga*
- Squash and squash blossoms
- Turmeric
- Turnips* and turnip greens*
- Yellow snapdragons

*Indicates sulforaphane-containing cruciferous vegetables.

Everything Else: Trace Minerals

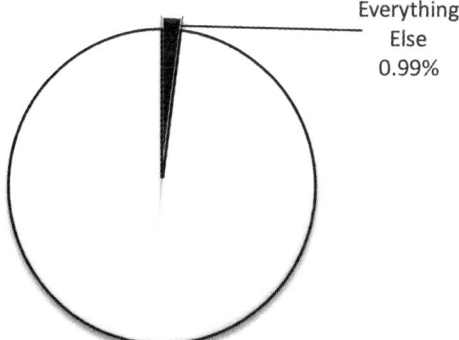

Everything Else 0.99%

The mass percent of "everything else" is 0.99 percent of your body's composition. This includes ten essential nutrients that make up a portion of the 0.99 percentage. Concerning these precious nutrient minerals the axiom, "good things come in small packages," certainly applies.

> **10 Essential Nutrient Minerals in the "Everything Else" Category:**
> - Chlorine
> - Cobalt
> - Copper
> - Iodine
> - Iron
> - Magnesium
> - Manganese
> - Molybdenum
> - Sodium
> - Zinc

Most of these ten nutrient minerals are considered micro-minerals because your body's daily requirement for them is less than 100 mg (milligrams). These nutrient micro-minerals work synergistically with one or more of their compatriots. It is of utmost importance that we have a sufficient supply and a precisely balanced formulation of these nutrient minerals. Nutrient micro-minerals participate in numerous metabolic processes and blood cell building, and they contribute to the structural integrity of many different tissues in your body.

In brief, sodium, potassium and chlorine are considered to be electrolytes and are pivotal in maintaining proper function of nerves and muscles, most especially your heart's contractions. Each one of that triad must be balanced with the other two components for proper "electrical" function in your body.

Calcium, phosphorus and magnesium are another triad of essential nutrient minerals that work together for building and maintaining strong bones and other body structures if they are properly balanced. Very small amounts of fluorine (natural calcium fluoride, not toxic sodium fluoride)[10], zinc, nickel, boron and silicon also contribute to proper bone and connective tissue growth and maintenance. A tiny amount of copper is helpful for bone, blood, hair and skin formation. A copper deficiency may be related to certain birth defects. Chromium, zinc and vanadium all work together to assist your blood sugar balance. Most people with hypoglycemia or diabetes find significant benefit from adding these healthful minerals in addition to eliminating processed foods and added sugars.

Magnesium is critically important for assisting in regulating your heart's rhythm. In addition, magnesium is an important co-enzyme and participates in more than 300 critical biochemical processes in your body every day. Both chocolate and dark leafy greens are rich in magnesium. It's interesting that more people seem to crave chocolate than crave a nice luscious bowl of Swiss chard or kale. Each chlorophyll molecule has an atom of magnesium in the center, while a similarly shaped molecule of hemoglobin (the oxygen-carrying molecule in your blood) only differs from chlorophyll by having an iron atom in the center.

> **Magnesium for Relaxation**
> A relaxing way to add magnesium to your system is to luxuriate in a hot Epsom salt bath, or to massage magnesium oil into your sore or spasming muscles. Refer to page 353 in *Your Body Can Talk, 2nd Edition* to discover resources regarding magnesium flakes and magnesium oil.

Twelve other trace elements are considered highly beneficial to the body, but are not currently considered essential. These trace elements, when supplied in their proper amount, may contribute to health, wellness and increased tissue strength. You may be shocked to read the names of a few of these, like arsenic and lead for instance, since you likely associate them with being toxic or poisonous. As we learn more about the human body and its needs, we are finding that even arsenic and lead (in the appropriate **tiny** amounts) may play important and even health promoting roles. However, in an amount above the tiny beneficial quantity, many of these trace elements are toxic or even lethal.

Beneficial Trace Elements

• Arsenic	• Fluorine	• Selenium
• Boron	• Lead	• Silicon
• Cadmium	• Lithium	• Tin
• Chromium	• Nickel	• Vanadium

Since a tiny difference in quantity can make such a dramatic and life-impacting difference, trace mineral evaluation does not qualify as a do-it-yourself endeavor. You may need to add certain trace minerals, or detoxify from an excess or even a toxic amount of specific elements such as lead, iron, copper, fluorine, arsenic, cadmium or nickel. In this case, it is much safer to rely on your trusted healthcare practitioner, medical doctor, Clinical Kinesiologist or nutritionist. In some instances, specific testing of blood, urine, or hair will reveal an important secret about a minute mineral imbalance that may make all the difference in your health.

Other Useful Trace Minerals
- Arsenic, in very small amounts may deter breast cancer and leukemia, but in excessive amounts it promotes many other cancers, and can function as a fatal poison.
- Cobalt is an integral part of vitamin B_{12} (methylcobalamin).
- Copper, in a tiny amount, is helpful for bone, blood, hair and skin formation.
- Iodine is required for your thyroid hormone production and may prevent cancer, especially breast and prostate.
- Iron is utilized within your red blood cells to make hemoglobin and move oxygen through your body.
- Manganese strengthens your ligaments and should be supplemented when you are healing from a sprain.
- Selenium is critical for your immune function. It also teams up with Vitamin E and strengthens the heart muscle and protects you from cancer.
- Zinc also builds your immune system by specifically strengthening the spleen and thymus gland.

VITAMINS

> **Elements:** All vitamins contain carbon and hydrogen. Either oxygen or nitrogen (or both) are constituent elements of each vitamin. Certain vitamins also contain an additional specific element such as cobalt, phosphorus or sulfur.
>
> **Biological Purpose:** Vitamins participate in your body's ability to use other nutrients. They function as a catalyst and/or a regulator for metabolism, digestion and absorption.
>
> **Biochemical Classification:** Organic (contains carbon that defines living organisms)
>
> **Food Energy Potential:** 0 Calories, not a source of food energy
>
> **Required Enzymes:** Fat-soluble vitamins require lipase. (Food containing any vitamin must be properly digested to release the vitamin into your system.)

To supply necessary vitamins to our bodies we depend on our robust diet of healthy and natural unprocessed foods, and for most of us the addition of pure and natural vitamin supplements. Vitamins are essential to healthy and youthful living. For example, an ample supply of vitamin C is necessary for your body to produce the collagen that helps maintain skin texture and firmness. Perhaps you have seen a person who has been a heavy smoker for decades who has exaggerated wrinkling and sagging of their skin. Smoking depletes your body's short-term supply of vitamin C. In this case the person did not resupply vitamin C sufficiently before the next cigarette.

> **Vitamin Deficiency**
> - A deficiency of any individual vitamin can result in a specific deficiency disease.
> - Chronic vitamin A deficiency can cause night blindness and the diminishment of visual acuity.
> - A B_6 deficiency can result in anemia or peripheral neuropathy (pain or sensory disturbance of the feet and legs and/or hands and arms.)
> - The classic vitamin C deficiency is scurvy, characterized by excessive bruising and bleeding. Bleeding of the gums and loosening of the teeth also result from vitamin C deficiency. Anemia and weakened immunity are also potential consequences of vitamin C deficiency.
> - Vitamin B_9 or folate (sometimes referred to as folic acid) deficiency can cause anemia and nerve dysfunction.

> **Alcohol: The Anti-vitamin**
> Alcoholic beverages destroy or deactivate vitamins. This is partially responsible for the "hangover headache" and why some people try to prevent it with extra B-vitamin complex. Obviously, the less stressful solution for your body is to moderate or avoid alcohol. Excessive alcohol intake can diminish fat-soluble vitamins and wash them out of your system. This helps explain why longterm alcohol abuse seems to age a person far beyond their years.

B_{12}, the Youthing Vitamin: Every Elder's Friend

Because our ability to absorb vitamin B_{12} diminishes as we age, many elders feel remarkably more energetic when they supplement with methylcobalamin. It is the most pertinent vitamin for us to discuss. This form of vitamin B_{12} helps your entire body, including most of your metabolic functions, your digestion, repair, growth and development of all cells, as well as all of your nervous system and nerve functions throughout your life. Vitamin B_{12} helps your body to detoxify itself from many naturally occurring biochemical byproducts.

> **Vitamin B_{12} Deficiency Signs and Symptoms**
> 1. Anemia (possibly associated with other nutrients such as folate)
> 2. Neurological signs and symptoms
>   Irritability and mood swings and anxiety, fatigue, depression, confusion and cognitive decline (even atrophy of the brain). Poor balance, sleep issues and restless leg syndrome may be consequences of vitamin B_{12} deficiency. Lack of Vitamin B_{12} may contribute to insomnia and sleep issues.
> 3. Symmetrical neurological symptoms
>   Paresthesias consisting of numbness, tingling, and/or prickly sensations in the extremities. This can manifest in hands and arms and/or feet and legs.
> 4. Whole body signs and symptoms
>   Impaired immunity and increased susceptibility to colds and infections. Weakness and/or soreness of the limbs. Constipation or other bowel disturbances and increased heart disease risk.

Vitamin B_{12} is plentifully supplied in most meat and dairy foods. Anyone who routinely includes meat (especially liver), poultry, fish or shellfish in their diet several times a week is likely accessing B_{12} consistently. Lacto-ovo vegetarians who include dairy products and eggs are also receiving vitamin B_{12} when consuming those foods; however, there is some evidence that cooking eggs reduces the amount of available B_{12}. Those who are consistently consuming a vegan diet are typically advised to take a vitamin B_{12} supplement. The online journal *Nutrients* has published a fairly comprehensive look at plant-based vitamin B_{12} sources.[11]

YOUR BODY'S MACRONUTRIENTS

The second category of essential nutrients is macronutrients. This group includes proteins, carbohydrates and fats. Each type of macronutrient provides your body with healthful nutrition and fuel, especially when consumed in an unadulterated or unprocessed form.

Avocados, almonds and farm-raised eggs are well-balanced and contain all of the macronutrients. I consider each of these to be "perfect foods" because they have protein, carbohydrate and fat. Aside from allergy and sensitivity issues, these are good to include in your diet, especially at breakfast. Too often, people have a breakfast of processed (and therefore nutrient poor) carbohydrates with added sugar. Adding wholesome sources of fat and protein will balance your blood sugar and prime your metabolism to operate efficiently throughout the day. Eating half or even a whole avocado with a spoon, or putting it in your smoothie will go far to satisfy your need for a morning dose of healthy fat and protein.[12]

I often slice an organic apple into wedges, arrange them on a small plate, and spread almond butter on one end of each piece. This provides a simple and easy-to-digest source of unaltered carbohydrate, protein and fat. Adding these and similar food combinations into your youthing lifestyle may help avert midmorning headaches or feeling famished just before lunch.

Proteins and Amino Acids

> **Proteins**
> **Composed of:** various amino acids
> **Elements:** Carbon, Hydrogen, Oxygen, Nitrogen and Sulfur.
> **Approximate percentage of body weight:** 17 percent
> **Biological Purpose:** growth and repair of tissues
> **Food Energy Potential:** 4 Calories/gram
> **Required Enzymes (most basic):** Proteases

Dietary proteins are available from both the plant and animal kingdoms. Whether or not a person chooses to select from both of these kingdoms is a personal choice. By using sprouts, nuts, seeds, legumes and grains it is possible to assure your necessary protein intake if you choose to be vegan or vegetarian. It is wise to be well educated on this topic and to seek nutritional counsel if you are uncertain about your dietary choices. The most important aspect of your protein intake should be that it is a pure, natural and unadulterated source that your body can fully digest and benefit from.

Proteins are the most difficult of the macronutrients to digest and many people above the age of forty require supplemental digestive enzymes to effectively digest protein. Digestive enzymes are not traditionally considered an essential nutrient because the human body (albeit well-nourished and younger than forty) produces digestive enzymes on a daily basis. Supplemental digestive enzymes should be added to our list of helpful and health-promoting nutritional supplements. In order to avoid a possible downward spiral that will occur without simple supplemental intervention, I recommend that you evaluate your personal need for digestive enzyme supplements by using Clinical Kinesiology testing. Refer to pages xvii-xviii in the Introduction to review the testing procedure.

A simple Kinesiology test can be accomplished by holding some concentrated protein—whether it's dry beans, fresh sprouts, shelled nuts or an egg—in your hand, and using a Clinical Kinesiology test for compatibility. By doing these simple muscle tests, you can learn a lot of valuable information. If any of the items selected test weak, hold the food item plus a digestive enzyme and retest. If the food was first weak but then strengthens with the presence of the enzyme, you may consider that the combination is compatible with your body. It is best to check several different protein sources and more than one enzyme selection.

If you are going to use a protein powder or protein supplement be selective, and choose only from the highest quality products. If you use a protein supplement, non-denatured whey may suit your needs. Vegans can use a rice-based or pea-based protein supplement. The potential problem with any of these products is often over processing, the addition of refined sugar and lack of bioavailability. I generally use an unsweetened and bio-available combination of whey and sprouted organic vegetables; sometimes I substitute this with a ground Brazil nut protein powder that has nothing added or removed.

> **Amino Acids for Longevity (Often Added as Supplemental Nutrients)**
> - L-carnitine helps our bodies to turn fat into energy and has been shown to strengthen the heart muscle and assist with most types of cardiac issues. It may also help to normalize blood sugar and blood fats and even aid in the relief of extreme fatigue and depression.
> - Acetyl L-carnitine helps preserve or improve brain and memory function. It may help lower heart rate and help muscle function. It is known to mend and bolster telomeres.
> - L-carnosine is a cleansing and detoxifying agent that helps your body remove heavy metals, toxic metals and debris of broken down cells and biochemicals. It also acts as a rejuvenator for many body areas such as skin, vascular system, nerve tissues and even internal organs. It is known to mend and bolster telomeres.
> - Serine helps the brain and central nervous system to function more efficiently.
> - Tryptophan assures you a sufficient supply of serotonin and helps you to maintain contentment and a positive mood.

> **Proteins That Your Body Must Build Every Day**
> - Antibodies that are key components for your immune system function
> - Contractile proteins (actin and myosin) that allow for muscle contractions and allow you to practice your Essentrics, Tai Chi, or tennis.

- Some enzymes are digestive enzymes, but many others function as catalysts for countless numbers of necessary biochemical reactions and processes in your body.
- Hormonal proteins such as insulin (transports and regulates your use of glucose, your body's primary fuel) and somatotropin (regulates protein synthesis in your muscles)
- Structural proteins that form the latticework for most of your bodily structures such as bones, hair, ligaments and even your organs. Examples of structural proteins include collagen, elastin and keratin.

It is easy to understand why your protein consumption is important. If your protein intake is insufficient or if you cannot break down and then repurpose your dietary proteins, the results may include loss of muscle tissue, degradation of your organs and saggy skin.

Carbohydrates

Elements: carbon, hydrogen, oxygen (usually in 2:1 ratio of hydrogen: oxygen, the same ratio as water).
Approximate percentage of body weight: 1.5 percent
Biological purpose: Primary energy source for body activities such as movement and brain and nerve function. Carbohydrates are energy packages and provide a mechanism to transport or store their useable energy, as well as transport vitamins and minerals into your body.
Food Energy Potential: 4 Calories/gram
Required Enzymes (most basic): Amylases

Carbohydrates are the most immediate and usable source of energy for our muscles, nerves and brain. The best way to think of carbohydrates is to consider that a food is a worthy and nutritious carbohydrate source if it was grown on or in a non-GMO and chemical-pesticide-free farm, garden, or orchard. The second qualifier is that the fruit, vegetable or nut looks like the real thing and still has its natural water content. In other words, the carbohydrates we will be discussing are actual unprocessed sources of energy and nutrients.

> **Disqualified Carbs**
> Carbohydrates that will be disqualified from our discussion and from a youthing-focused diet are typically in a box, package, vending machine, soft drink dispenser or can, or bakery case. You will have to use very little discernment to quickly recognize that the items just described do not look as if they grew on a farm, or tree, or in a garden. These are the culprits that have sullied the term "carbohydrates" for all those innocent and willing-to-nourish, true carbohydrates. May the real (and unprocessed) carbohydrates of the world forever take back their good reputation and their name!

Plant life is the primary source for carbohydrates. Plants, generally fruits, vegetables and nuts are largely composed of carbohydrates in a variety of forms. It is necessary for a human to consume significant portions of unprocessed and hopefully raw carbohydrates daily to provide his or her body with sufficient fuel for its functions and to obtain vitamins and minerals.

Many dietary plans suggest that forty-five to fifty-five percent of a person's dietary intake be in the form of carbohydrates. An unfortunate impediment to this ideal of consumption is that the terminology regarding carbs is ambiguous and changes from decade to decade.

The problem with refined and processed carbohydrates is that a more concentrated amount of sugars are added to processed foods and beverages. This causes the primitive areas of the human brain and consciousness to mistakenly accept these as healthy and non-toxic. We are programmed to seek out the sweet flavor, but it's best to trust nature and not to try to fool our taste buds with processed foods. The fructose in your apple or your green peas is in a stable and balanced context and has many other useful and synergistic nutrients present.

Lipids (Fats)

> **Elements:** carbon, hydrogen, oxygen
> **Approximate percentage of body weight:** 13.8 percent
> **Biological purpose:** Fats contribute to cell membrane structure giving stability. Nerve sheath coverings require fats and cholesterol in particular. Fats insulate and protect organs and tissues including the brain, nerves, eyes and skin. Fats are more than twice as effective as proteins and carbohydrates in storing energy. A very important function of fats is that they are both the carrier and storage medium for your fat-soluble vitamins (A, D, E and K).
> **Distinct biochemical property:** Fats are **not** soluble in water and are soluble in alcohol.
> **Food energy potential:** 9 Calories/gram.
> **Required Enzymes (most basic):** Lipases

Roughly ninety-five percent of the lipid content of our body is in triglyceride form—stored fat. Dietary fats are essential to human and mammalian life. Seventy percent of your brain's weight can be attributed to fat content. Fats are highly concentrated in certain food sources (typically meat and dairy-based), yet are surprisingly prevalent in unexpected plant sources. For instance, cauliflower contains brain protective and health promoting omega three fatty acids.

> ### Oils, the Bad and the Good
> Several commercially produced vegetable oils are sourced from Genetically Modified Organism (GMO) plants and contain trans fats, chemically modified fats. Please avoid these vegetable oils and the processed foods that they are literally poured into. They can be carcinogenic and deserve a bad rap. Prime examples are soy oil, canola oil, corn oil and cottonseed oil. Because most vegetable oils have been through one or more chemical or biological processes,

> and have an extremely high level of omega 6 essential fatty acids (that promote inflammation), the most logical step is to avoid these items to the best of your ability. Coconut oil, on the other hand, has been shown to be heart and cardiovascular protective, immune building, and helpful in blood sugar regulation. Bruce Fife, N.D., regarded as today's coconut oil expert, has written over twenty books on the topic, including: *Coconut Cure; The Coconut Oil Miracle; The Coconut Ketogenic Diet, Supercharge Your Metabolism, Revitalize Thyroid Function and Lose Excess Weight* and *Stop Alzheimer's Now!* I highly recommend reading one or more of Dr. Fife's books so that you can truly understand the safety and health protective nature of adding non-hydrogenated coconut oil to your diet.

Besides being heart healthy and anti-inflammatory (except in the case of excess Omega 6 fatty acids), unprocessed fat in your healthy food sources helps with skin and hair texture, assists in stabilizing your blood sugar and provides a feeling of satiety or fullness that in the long run may reduce your Caloric intake.

All of these essential nutrients, and others that have not been listed here, interact in multiple biochemical, metabolic, and hormonal chemical reactions that are occurring 24/7 within your body. All of your nutrients need to be sufficiently supplied and properly balanced with each other to impart health and longevity.

Water, Etc.
In addition to the nutrients just discussed, we all require water, air, sunlight, and lifestyle nutrients like adequate sleep and rest. These nutrients are often overlooked.

Water is the first to consider. Obviously the intake of clean and pure water is a requisite for all human and animal life. Your body composition is between fifty and seventy-five percent water (hydrogen and oxygen). It is interesting to note that the Earth's oceans, lakes, rivers and glaciers account for approximately seventy-five percent of the Earth's surface.

Most of us could improve our health, our body composition and our physiology by drinking more clean, pure water. Finding this high-quality water may be a bit frustrating. Especially if your typical water source is from a municipal supply, your best choice will be to search for the best water purification and filtration system you can find. Tap water is treated with a variety of chemicals, including chloramine, a chemical agent that combines chlorine and ammonia, and fluoride in the form of fluorosilicic acid and sodium fluoride. While these chemical additives have been deemed safe in tapwater by the United States Center of Disease Control and Prevention, many studies have shown these chemicals to be toxic and carcinogenic.

Water helps transport nutrients and normal biological chemicals (natural hormones, enzymes and immunity factors) throughout your body. It aids your nutrient absorption and therefore your overall health. It also plumps your skin, making it appear softer, smoother and less wrinkled.

Including fresh air, safe sunlight exposure, and proper rest and sleep round out a wise youthing lifestyle.

Live More, Eat Less
The quality of your food intake has been addressed, now a brief word about quantity. Okinawan tradition is to drink hot tea throughout the day and to say "hara hachi bu" just before each meal. This Confucian maxim means "eat until you are eighty-percent full." The Okinawans may be the only human population that purposefully restricts how many Calories they eat. Modern science has proven Calorie reduction to be a sure-fire life-extension method.

YOUR NUTRITIONAL BOTTOM-LINE
For A Youthing Lifestyle

> **Include:**
> 1. Eat a widely diverse roster of healthful unprocessed food. Change it up often.

Include:
2. Select foods sourced from growers and producers using "clean" growing practices and chemical-free methods.
3. Choose foods sourced from organic farms, orchards, ranches, dairies and gardens.
4. Look for GMO-free certified foods.
5. Select unadulterated foods (they look like they were just picked), chemical-free, preservative-free and additive-free.
6. Choose fruits and vegetables from the rainbow of natural colors: red, orange, yellow green, blue and purple, etc. This will give you a variety of healthy phytochemicals and extra vitamins and minerals.
7. Emphasize plant food categories including: fruits, vegetables (leafy and root). Use them in their raw forms frequently. Prepare vegetable and root dishes by steaming on the stovetop, baking, oven-roasting or cooking in a slow cooker.
8. Healthy fruits include: apples, apricots, avocados, blueberries, cantaloupe, citrus, kiwi, peaches, pineapple, raspberries, strawberries and watermelon. Broaden your choices and look for unusual and exotic fruits as well.
9. Healthy vegetables include: asparagus, beets, broccoli, carrots, dandelion greens, garlic, green beans, Jerusalem artichoke, kale, onions, peas, radishes, sweet potatoes, Swiss chard, turnips and various dark green salad greens. Choose from a wide variety and rotate your choices frequently.
10. Include healthy (preferably home-made) fermented foods such as live-culture sauerkraut (avoid versions that are canned or have added vinegar because there are no live probiotics in these), many other fermented vegetables, miso, yogurt and kefir.[13]
11. Raw nuts, raw seeds and dried seaweed. Prepare by soaking and draining before use.
12. Quinoa is actually a seed and provides high-quality protein. After rinsing well, cook on stovetop for twenty to thirty min-

Include:

utes, or in a slow-cooker for one to two hours. Use at least two cups of purified water per one cup of dry quinoa. Use at any meal with a medley of vegetables.

13. Mushrooms are a valuable protein source. You can sauté them in butter or coconut oil in large batches and store them in a sealed canning-type jar in your refrigerator (for up to one week). Add portions of the sautéed mushrooms to scrambled eggs, soups, stews, mixed vegetable dishes, etc.
14. Beans and legumes:
    a. If purchased in dry form, soak overnight, rinse and slow cook appropriately.
    b. You may also choose to sprout the beans or legumes for three days before eating raw on salads or as a garnish.
15. Unaltered healthy fat sources include coconut milk, coconut oil, organic whole milk dairy products from grass-fed or pasture-raised cows and goats. These may include butter, cheese, yogurt, cottage cheese, etc.
16. Organic, free-range, or organic pasture-raised eggs are the cleanest and most nutritious eggs.
17. If you eat meats, foul, or fish, use the criterion from numbers one through four above.
18. Whole, non-GMO, organic Grains (minimize their use). Choose varieties that provide a strong muscle test result. These are most friendly to your body when used in sprouted form.
19. Heartily drink the purest water you can find. Consider spring water, artesian well water or filtered and purified water.
20. Use your spring or purified and filtered water to make a variety of simple herbal teas with no additives.
21. Whenever possible, use glass containers for food storage.

Exclude:
1. A limited lackluster diet without variety
2. Processed and packaged foods
3. Food preservatives and additives such as: artificial sweeteners, BHA, BHT, diacetyl (artificial butter flavoring in microwave popcorn), emulsifiers, flavor enhancers, food dyes, high fructose corn sweetener or syrup, mono- and diglycerides, MSG, nitrates, nitrites, potassium bromate, sugar, sulfates, sulfides, sulfur dioxide and the like. Most of these cause significant health problems and many of them are considered carcinogenic.
4. Cured meats that contain nitrates or nitrites
5. Commercial-grade cage- or barn-raised or GMO-grain-fed eggs, dairy, and meats. The health of these animals may be compromised by their living conditions and food, and the resulting products may be of lesser nutritional quality.
6. Dairy, eggs, meat and poultry that had hormone injections or hormones added into the animal's feed
7. GMO foods or suspected GMO foods (no required labeling)
8. A grain- and flour-predominant diet
9. Sodas
10. Sugary beverages and sweetened juices
11. Fast foods and junk foods
12. Oils that are hydrogenated, partially hydrogenated or heat processed
13. Unfiltered tap-water (potentially containing chloramine, sodium fluoride, medication residues and chemical residues)
14. Styrofoam (polystyrene) packaging, storage, and food containers for foods and beverages. This includes the hard version of polystyrene that is most commonly found as plastic eating utensils, cups, and storage containers. Polystyrene is a known carcinogen and has been shown to leach out of food containers, especially when they are exposed to heat. Products composed of polystyrene contain the recycling symbol with a number 6 inside.
15. Excessive servings of coffee and black tea

> **Exclude:**
> 16. Excessive alcoholic beverage intake
>
> Refer back to and reread this chapter often. It can serve as a basic guide to understanding your body and the elements and components that form it. On a daily basis you should consider the ingredients and constituents of your foods and beverages. Remember to "eat what you are made of."

LEARN MORE

- Read Chapter 5, "Food and Energy" (pages 93-111) in *Your Body Can Talk, 2nd Edition* by Susan L. Levy, D.C. for an understanding of how foods are compatible with your body.
- GMO Foods and their problems are discussed on pages 96-98 and 103 in *Your Body Can Talk, 2nd Edition* by Susan L. Levy, D.C.
- To learn more about fermented foods, read pages 154-156 in *Your Body Can Talk, 2nd Edition* by Susan L. Levy, D.C.

Books

Adams, Mike. *Food Forensics: The Hidden Toxins Lurking in Your Food and How You Can Avoid Them for Lifelong Health*. Dallas, Texas: BenBella Books, Inc., 2016

Braverman, Eric R., M.D. *The Healing Nutrients Within*. North Bergen, New Jersey: Basic health Publications, 2003.

Cohen, Suzy, RPh. *Drug Muggers: Which Medications Are Robbing Your Body of Essential Nutrients--and Natural Ways to Restore Them*. New York: Rodale Books, 2011.

Di Justo, Patrick. *This is What You Just Put in Your Mouth?: From Eggnog to Beef Jerky, the Surprising Secrets*. New York: Three Rivers Press, 2015.

Fife, Bruce, N.D. *The Coconut Oil Miracle, 5th Edition*. New York: Avery Publishing, 2013.

Fife, Bruce, N.D. *The Coconut Ketogenic Diet: Supercharge Your Metabolism, Revitalize Thyroid Function and Lose Excess Weight*. Colorado Springs, Colo.: Piccadilly Books, Ltd., 2014.

Enig, Mary and Sally Fallon. *Eat Fat, Lose Fat: The Healthy Alternative to Trans Fats.* New York: Hudson Street Press, 2006.

Kliment, Felicia. *The Acid Alkaline Balance Diet, Second Edition: An Innovative Program that Detoxifies Your Body's Acidic Waste to Prevent Disease and Restore Overall Health.* New York: The McGraw-Hill Companies, 2010.

Lipman, Frank, M.D. *10 Reasons You Feel Old and Get Fat: And How you Can Stay Young, Slim and Happy!* Carlsbad, Calif.: Hay House, Inc., 2016.

Smith, Jeffrey. *Genetic Roulette: The Documented Health Risks of Genetically Engineered Foods.* Fairfield, Iowa: Yes! Books, 2007.

Yiamouyiannis, John. *Fluoride the Aging Factor: How to Recognize and Avoid the Devastating Effects of Fluoride, 3rd Edition.* Ohio: Health Action Press, 1993.

Websites

Farm to Consumer Legal Defense Fund: www.farmtoconsumer.org/)
Campaign for Real Milk: www.realmilk.com
Fermented Foods and Probiotics: https://www.youtube.com/watch?v=P-DdD_P1_5k

Products

3Sixty5™ for Adults Multivitamin: http://mymangosteen.com/DrSusan/product/3SIXTY5.asp

Dreaming Cow Plain, Whole Milk Yogurt (grass fed, no sugar or additives): http://www.dreamingcow.com/

Favao™ Protein Powder: http://mymangosteen.com/DrSusan/product/favao_protein.asp

Food Matters T.V. Health and Wellness programming online: https://www.fmtv.com/join-today

Kerrygold® Grass-Fed Butter and Cheese: http://www.kerrygoldusa.com/

Maple Hill Creamery® Plain, Whole Milk Yogurt (grass fed, no sugar or additives): http://maplehillcreamery.com/creamontop-plain.html

Native Forest Organic Classic, Unsweetened Coconut Milk: http://www.edwardandsons.com/native_shop_coconut.itml

Piix™ Digestion Tincture: http://mymangosteen.com/DrSusan/product/piix_digestion.asp

Straus Family Creamery™ Organic, Plain, Whole Milk Yogurt (grass fed, no sugar or additives): http://strausfamilycreamery.com/products/item/organic-plain-yogurt

T.J. Clark, Original Colloidal Mineral Formula: http://tjclark.net/tjcoriginal.htm

Vital Farms® Pasture-Raised eggs: http://vitalfarms.com/pasture-raised-eggs/

Xalo® Ageless: http://mymangosteen.com/DrSusan/product/XALO_Ageless.asp

Xalo® Ignite: http://mymangosteen.com/DrSusan/product/xalo_ignite.asp

Xalo® Limitless: http://mymangosteen.com/DrSusan/product/xalo_limitless.asp

Xalo® Reload: http://mymangosteen.com/DrSusan/product/xalo_reload.asp

Xango® Juice: http://mymangosteen.com/DrSusan/product/juice_xango.asp

Endnotes, Chapter 5

1. Smith, Jeffrey. *Genetic Roulette: The Documented Health Risks of Genetically Engineered Foods.* Fairfield, Iowa: Yes! Books, 2007.
2. Braverman, Eric R., M.D. *The Healing Nutrients Within.* North Bergen, New Jersey: Basic Health Publications, 2003.
3. Cohen, Suzy, RPh. *Drug Muggers: Which Medications Are Robbing Your Body of Essential Nutrients—and Natural Ways to Restore Them.* New York: Rodale Books, 2011. 115-118.
4. Calvo, Mona S. and Katherine L. Tucker. "Is Phosphorus Intake that Exceeds Dietary Requirements a Risk Factor in Bone Health?" *ANNALS of the New York Academy of Sciences*, 1301, 2013, 29-35.
5. Cohen, 74.
6. Boyles, Saylnn. "Stroke Rounds: Potassium Tied to Lower Stroke Rist." *MedPage Today.* Sept. 14, 2014. Accessed Feb. 26, 2016: http:www.medpagetoday.com/Geriatrics/GeneralGeriatrics/47497
7. Cohen, 224-226.

8   Zhang, Y. P. Talalay, C.G. Cho and G.H. Posner. "A Major Inducer of Anticarcinogenic Protective Enzymes from Broccoli: Isolation ad Elucidation of Structure." *Proceedings of the National Academy of Sciences of the United States of America*. 89:6 (March 1992): 2399-2403. http://www.ncbi.nlm.nih.gov/pmc/articles/PMC48665/. (accessed February 29,2016)
9   Benedict, Andrea L., Andrea Mountney, Andres Hurtado, Kelley E. Bryan, Ronald L. Schnaar, Albena T. Dinkova-Kostova and Paul Talalay. " Neuroprotective Effects of Sulforaphane after Contusive Spinal Cord Injury." *Journal of Neurotrauma*. 29: 16 (November 1, 2012): 2576-2586. http://www.ncbi.nlm.nih.gov/pmc/articles/PMC3495118/ (accessed February 29, 2016).
10 Yiamouyiannis, John. *Fluoride the Aging Factor: How to Recognize and Avoid the Devastating Effects of Fluoride, 3rd Edition*. Ohio: Health Action Press, 1993.
11 Watanabe, Fumio, Yukinori Yabuta, Tomohiro Bito, and Fei Teng. "Vitamin B12 Containing Plant Food Sources for Vegetarians." *Nutrients*. 6:5 (2014). 1861-1873
12 Fulgoini III, Victor L., Mark Dreher and Adrienne J. Davenport. "Avocado Consumption is Associated with Better Diet Quality and Nutrient Intake, and Lower Metabolic Syndrome Risk in US Adults: Results from the National Health and Nutrition Examination Survey (NHANES) 2001-2008." *Nutrition Journal*. 12:1 (January 2, 2013). http://nutritionj.biomedcentral.com/articles/10.1186/1475-2891-12-1 (accessed March 12, 2016).
13 Levy, Susan L. D.C., *Your Body Can Talk, 2nd Edition*. Chino Valley, Ariz.: Kalindi Press, 2014. 154-156.

CHAPTER 6

... and Trash the Rest: Detoxing for Longevity

Take a moment to visualize a small aquarium containing two goldfish. Now let's imagine that it is your job to care for these fish and keep them not only alive, but optimally functioning. Your responsibilities will include providing safe and appropriate water, at an optimal temperature. Quality food sources, air supply, sunshine and cleanliness are also necessary. For our purposes in considering the subject of detoxification, think of your individual cells, the most basic biological building blocks of your body, as individual goldfish within their own small aquariums.

Since your goldfish are captive in this aquarium and cannot escape to search for more optimal conditions, you the caretaker are entrusted with consistently obtaining and providing clean and pure water. Since tap water contains chloramine or chlorine, your first responsibility will be to remove or neutralize these chemicals. Chloramine, effective for killing single-celled organisms, is added to municipal water supplies and many domestic wells as a disinfectant to kill bacteria, algae and fungus. Chloramine can also be quite effective in killing your goldfish and even some of your own cells, not to mention killing the beneficial and vitally important bacteria in your intestinal tract. To remove chemicals, you can filter your fishes' water, and do the same for your drinking water.

More than once each day your goldfish will need to relieve themselves of biological wastes, thus dirtying and clouding their water, which is not only their immediate environment but the substance that sustains their lives. As with your pet goldfish, your own cells and your entire body are constantly utilizing and metabolizing nutrients as well as rapidly producing significant amounts of toxic-waste byproducts. These need to be eliminated expediently from both your fishes' and your cell's tissue and cellular fluids.

Certainly you will change the water in the aquarium frequently so that your goldfish will not have to struggle in toxic, turbid water. The advantage that the goldfish have is that any observer will immediately notice the dirty water that needs to be changed. The disadvantage that your cells experience is that their cellular fluids are invisible, and so their needs may be ignored. Two helpful hints for us humans will be to drink sufficient (even copious) amounts of fresh purified water, and to undertake specific detoxification or cleansing measures frequently.

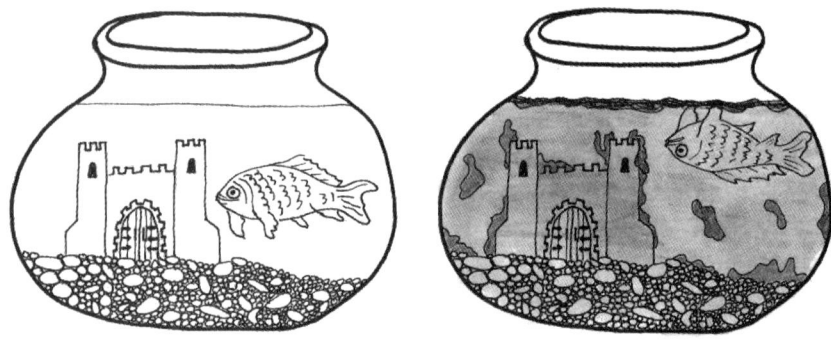

As curator of both your aquarium and your own body's cells, you will need to provide for appropriate shelter, temperature, unadulterated fresh and healthy pure foods, a continuous supply of clean water, as well as sufficient clean air and appropriate sunlight. A healthy environment for a small unit of life, either a goldfish or a human cell, will obviously have other important requirements, such as a calm atmosphere and a feeling of safety.

Let's examine how easily your cells are exposed to toxins and how you can begin to detoxify your body.

TOXINS

"How did the toxins get into my cells and my body?" you may ask. But you may not like the answer: You probably let most of them in yourself.

An estimated 600,000 toxic substances occur in our environment. Since we are chemically akin to our immediate environment, as we pollute the air, water and soils of the earth, we cannot help but absorb those same foreign toxins directly into our own body along with the important and essential nutrients we need to survive, like potassium and oxygen. Your responsibility as the proprietor of a wise and aging body intent on a richer, fuller life, lies in discovering more about these many toxins and how to avoid them when possible.

The vast majority of these toxins exist because of industrial waste, pharmaceutical pollution, chemically-based agriculture, certain types of energy production and the burning of fossil fuels. Toxins from those sources are found in the air, water and soil. They are in many products that you bring into your home, including textiles, building materials, medications, cleaning agents, cosmetics, body care products, food additives, and packaged or processed "foods."

As we saw in the metaphor that began this chapter, tap water may contain problematic pollutants such as chloramine. It also may contain harmful residues from medications that have been flushed down the toilet and reenter your local water system. Municipal water purification plants are typically not sophisticated enough to filter out these complicated chemical toxins. By avoiding the drinking of tap water, or at least filtering it sufficiently, you can eliminate unwanted doses of someone else's medications.

While it is a bit daunting, do not be completely discouraged by all the potential sources of toxicity around you. Working to avoid them will require some effort, however. The most reasonable approach is to select detoxification principles and procedures that you can easily live with. The first principle is to **limit your exposure to toxins wherever and whenever possible**.

Consuela's Story

Consuela was miserable. She had known that she had a serious degree of lactose intolerance and suspected that she had celiac disease for a number of years. She had modified her diet with those considerations, but still felt terrible. As each year of her life passed, she felt that she had aged two or three years. Consuela had a long list of inflammatory symptoms and a number of problematic health conditions. Brain fog, poor memory and sporadic impaired judgment plagued her. Worst of all she had no stamina. In spite of being ill and having very low energy, Consuela rarely had a good night's sleep and was restless and miserable through most of every night.

During her exam I found Consuela had a significant level of heavy metal toxicity. She had a mouth full of amalgam (mercury-containing, silver-colored) dental fillings. She knew that she wanted these removed as soon as possible knowing that that was likely the key to her health problems. Her biological dentist and I both advised her to proceed gradually with the amalgam removal and subsequent dental restorations. Under this type of scenario, a patient generally needs intensive detoxification and healthcare support. Consuela was desperate to make a change and feel better. Her quality of life was at such a low ebb that she questioned the use of going on. All the fillings in her teeth were removed in a short period of time and replaced with nontoxic materials.

Consuela diligently took saunas at home and had Aqua Chi® cleansing footbath treatments in my office along with many other treatments and nutritional support. All of these measures ultimately contributed to helping detoxify Consuela's body, and reduced the toxic load. The ultimate goal was to reduce her total body toxicity. Once that was achieved, her level of inflammation diminished.

DETOXING YOUR HOME ENVIRONMENT

Working to improve the overall environment within your home, office and vehicle is a fairly easy step. A good place to begin is with your clothing, bedding, textiles, upholstery and carpeting. Organic materials (like cotton or hemp) used in fabrics do not harbor the residue of any pesticides used during the growing phase of these materials, nor other chemicals that could be used in the processing, weaving and sewing phases of fabric production. Fabrics that are not organic often outgas pollutants into the air of a home. If this outgassing occurs, you may absorb toxins through your skin, as well as breathe them into your lungs. Once toxins are inside your body, they move into your bloodstream and circulate throughout your system. Fortunately, organically-certified fabrics are becoming more popular and more available.

I recommend that you use organic textiles when possible to simplify your home detoxing process. Remember to launder new linens and clothing before use to further eliminate possible toxic residue. Use water-based carpet-cleaning processes, such as ZEROREZ® (see www.zerorez.com).

In general, consider properly disposing of chemical household cleansers, pesticides, cosmetics and other supplies, and scaling back to a bare-bones and all-natural selection of these items. Every toxic chemical substance you have can be replaced with a more natural alternative. You can even find natural pest-deterring essential oils, such as cedar oil, for use in your home and garden. Cedarcide® is a reputable and natural pest deterring product line.

A. Air

Controlling air quality in your indoor environment is an easily manageable task. Start with avoiding aerosol sprays, chemical compounds, bug sprays, hairspray, etc. Naturally, you have the right to declare your car, home or workplace as a cigarette and vape-free zone. I also recommend that you greatly minimize or eliminate the presence of toxic-chemical-based cleaning products in your home. Instead you can use simple, do-it-yourself cleaning agents such as a vinegar and water mixture. Other choices are commercially available, such as plain castile soap, or Dr. Bronner's liquid soap. Periodically cleaning and maintaining heat, air and ventilation duct-work will also prove beneficial.

> **Warning: Small Portable Home Humidifiers**
> These humidifiers, particularly the cool-mist type, are notorious for growing harmful mold or fungus colonies. I advise against these

units. If you feel you must use a cool-mist humidifier, I suggest you rotate two or three units on a daily basis. Once you use unit one for twenty-four hours or less, unplug it, empty it, sanitize it with vinegar or even Clorox®, rinse and leave it to dry for twenty-four or more hours. During this time, use unit two and/or three, never more than twenty-four hours each. One of my patients kept refilling the same unit that was in use continually for weeks. She did not notice the mucus-like, pale-colored slime in the bottom of the unit and became sick and incapacitated for weeks. She had to leave her home and convalesce at a relative's home.

If you invest in a whole-home humidification system, investigate thoroughly to be sure that no chance for microbial growth is possible in that unit.

Better Plan for Home Humidity
Boil water in a large uncovered pan on the stovetop occasionally.

The Power of Plants
Another "Better Plan" for increasing humidity in your home is to grow houseplants, water them appropriately (do not over water and promote fungus), and occasionally spray a light mist of water on them. Houseplants both clean and slightly moisten the air. Natural houseplants are living air filters. In particular, tropical bromeliads are known to filter toxins from room air. NASA researched the benefit of common houseplants on space missions. They discovered that astronauts benefited greatly.[1]

Forever Ban Formaldehyde
Most people would not knowingly bring formaldehyde into their home, but do so inadvertently. Formaldehyde may leach into your indoor air from Formica®, particle board, processed wood, furniture glue, mattresses, bed linens, clothing, curtains, shower

> curtains, and many plastic items. Some types of insulation (prior to 1982) were laden with formaldehyde.
>
> If your shampoo contains quaternium-15, you are massaging formaldehyde into your scalp and tresses regularly. This may explain headaches for some people.
>
> Avoiding formaldehyde in its many forms and combinations is essential to detoxification and health improvement. Opening and airing out your home daily, or at least every few days, will help eliminate persistent formaldehyde buildup.
>
> Strategically placing formaldehyde-filtering plants in your home, especially in your bedroom, is a pleasant and effective way to improve air quality in your home, and will help you in your quest for detoxification and cleaner living. For the cleansing of formaldehyde residue in room air, easily available plants such as: bamboo palm, Janet Craig, mother-in-law's tongue, and marginata are the best choices.[2] These and other plants can remove chemicals such as benzene and trichloroethylene (TCE) from your air as well.

In addition to beautiful plants, electric air filters, such as HEPA filters, and even bags of specialized charcoal can be helpful. The MoSo Bags® contain non-toxic, chemical- and fragrance-free bamboo charcoal.[3] Gonzo Odor Eliminator™ is a similar product, and is a bag containing highly absorbent volcanic rock. These products absorb various pollutants, including, allergens, mold spores and even excess moisture.

Each of us can have a small impact on outdoor air quality too, but for many of us this prospect may seem challenging. If you live in an already polluted area, or in one that is subject to periodic smog, you are encouraged to keep your body's internal environment as pure as possible by undergoing cleansing and detoxification regimens on a frequent basis. (These strategies will be covered later in this chapter.) Another tool for coping with the pollution surrounding you is to frequently visit a cleaner air site, which could be a wonderful getaway.

You can benefit from camping, boating, hiking, bicycling or horseback riding in a cleaner air region that is still easily accessible to you. If you are able to be in a forest of tall trees you can benefit directly from their expired oxygen. Spending time at the beach, near a stream of running water, a lake, or a reservoir will provide you with cleaner air, peace of mind and very likely sunshine as well.[4] If your local municipal botanical garden is more accessible to you, it will be a splendid and refreshing outing.

B. Detoxify Your Kitchen (and Your Diet)
Moving into your kitchen, your new "keep the toxins out" lifestyle, begins with a thorough assessment of your cabinets, your pantry and your refrigerator. Have a large trashcan ready so that you can detoxify your kitchen and rid yourself of chemically-laden or processed foods and condiments. You may even need two trash cans! It's time to seriously offload candy, cookies, pretzels, chips, high-heat treated vegetable oils, commercial grade salad dressings and all those items you may not want to talk about. Just get them out of your kitchen. If you are uncertain whether a certain item meets the qualifications of being pure and natural, unadulterated, non-GMO and hopefully organic, you can utilize your Clinical Kinesiology testing skills to determine if the item is compatible with your body. If your muscle response to the item is weak—trash it!

You may want to have a friend or relative or your Clinical Kinesiology practitioner double and triple check your findings about food choices. I recommend this because it is often difficult to remain emotionally neutral about certain foods, especially comfort foods or those you have an emotional attachment to.

Label reading is a fairly easy task; however, as label writing is sometimes convoluted or incomplete, you will need to do this carefully. Be alert for ingredients with chemical names, or names that you cannot pronounce. These items will often be the ones that add toxins to your system, impacting your health and potentially your longevity.

Once you have cleaned the kitchen of toxic food, you have come to a moment of truth. Will you do your best to keep it that way? I strongly recommend that you make a promise or a pledge to yourself (and to your kitchen) that, insofar as you are able, you will bring healthful and non-toxic foods, spices, teas and consumables into this freshly cleaned kitchen. If so, or simply to keep the motivation alive, you can write this principle on your message board: **My healthy kitchen is consistently full of healthy non-toxic foods.**

Detoxing your kitchen does not end with your food though. Glass cookware and storage containers are chemical free and are chemically inert, meaning that no residue from the container will enter your foods. You may choose to keep a variety of clean Mason-style jars and lids on hand to store staples and leftovers. Earthenware (verified to be lead-free) cookware, Crock-pots®, and enameled cast iron pots and pans do not leech anything into your food, unlike their "non-stick" counterparts. Toxic chemical residue is going to seep into your scrambled eggs and any other foods if you use a "non-stick" pan to cook them in.

While you are detoxing your kitchen by gathering up and tossing out your non-stick and your aluminum cookware and plastic food containers, I have another challenge for you. Will you also give a hearty heave to your radiation-producing, protein-denaturing microwave oven? I know that for many people this appliance has become integral to their way of life. But, do consider that it also poses health risks you certainly do not need. Instead, look for a toaster oven or a small countertop convection oven. Both are simple to use and to clean, and do not emit radiation.

With some or all of these recommendations set in place you will be making great strides toward a healthy diet and lifestyle. You are now prepared to engage in your most suitable diet as you eat "what you are made of," which is well described in Chapter 5.

INTERNAL DETOXING
Drink Up: The Importance Of Water
One of the easiest and most effective daily detoxification procedures is to liberally hydrate yourself with pure water. Water is the ultimate solvent and the best one to expose your body to. You should consistently be flushing your body with pure water every day.

A slight modification which augments cleansing is to squeeze the juice of one-half an organic lemon into about eight ounces of pure water and drink this in the morning before breakfast. The lemon juice adds minerals to your water, primes your digestion, and mildly nudges your liver to detoxify itself. I drink this organic lemon juice water early each morning and then take the skin of the lemon and cut that in smaller strips and rub the remaining lemon juice and pulp on my face, leaving it for a few minutes before washing with a toxin-free, organic cleanser. This clarifies the skin, helps maintain the normal skin pH and can help lighten discolored spots.

It is just as advisable to remove chloramine, chlorine and fluoride from your drinking water as it is for removing it from your goldfish's aquarium. I personally prefer the Berkey® water purification and filtration system to process my drinking water. It does a thorough job and is portable enough to take camping. The Berkey® Company also offers an optional arsenic and fluoride filter for their units. Multipure® is another effective water filter to consider. In my experience, inexpensive water filtration systems (under $300 or so) do not sufficiently filter water. Remember to store your water in glass, porcelain, or food-grade pottery containers.

> **Building a Clean Water System**
> If you are an avid do-it-yourselfer, you may want to read up on building your own atmospheric water generator at http://www.instructables.com/id/DIY-Atmospheric-Water-Generator/. These instructions guide you to build your own "make pure water from the humidity in air" machine for about $300. Commercial units begin at $1,200.00.

Juice Fasting for Internal Detox
Fresh-made juices from organic produce are cleansing and detoxifying while they bring a rich supply of micronutrients into your body. Periodic fasting is an effective cleansing technique, especially while you use fresh-made organic juices. Unless you have experience with juice

fasting, I recommend that you undertake this practice for the first time with your natural healthcare provider's approval and guidance. (See Kalindi Press, *The Detox Miracle Sourcebook*, by Robert S. Morse, N.D. for careful guidelines.) A cleansing juice fast usually lasts from three days to several weeks. It is quite a commitment, and requires preparation and planning because your diet must be modified and lightened both prior to beginning and at the end of the fast. However, adding fresh homemade juices are a wonderful addition to your pure and natural diet. (More about specific juices on pages 130-132.)

Most people "fast" every night before getting up to have breakfast, which actually means "break the fast." A simpler approach to fasting to support regular detoxing involves extending your nightly fast to give your body a little more downtime for doing its own internal cleansing. If you choose to have a mini-fast once or twice a week, or once or twice a month, you could simply skip a meal and extend your nighttime fasting.

A Mini-Fast Prescription

To undertake a safe, useful mini-fast, take a part of a day to prepare yourself. Start with breakfast in the morning of your fast. I advise people to always eat breakfast and to include at least one protein, carbohydrate and fat in this meal. Physiologically, breakfast is the most important meal of the day. But eating a breakfast that is lighter than normal would be an excellent way to prepare for your fast. Be sure to omit coffee, sugary orange juice and all those foods you've already committed to leave out of your dietary plan (see Chapter 5).

Hours later, have a nutritious light lunch, and then begin your mini-fast following lunch and through the night until the next morning.

Continue drinking greater-than-normal amounts of pure water during your fasting hours; or, you can include plain and simple herbal teas without extra flavorings or sweeteners. Yogi Tea® makes a tasty and effective detoxifying tea.

You should discuss this approach with your natural healthcare provider or nutritionist since you may have a special need or a condition that could contraindicate a mini fast of this type.

PERSONAL HYGIENE AND DETOXING

Your skin is your largest organ, also your largest organ of elimination. As you perspire, your body releases toxins (that are easily washed off). Few people stop to consider that their skin pores also allow toxins *inside* their body. The numerous toxic chemicals in typical skin lotions, deodorants, cosmetics and sunscreens easily enter your skin's pores after you simply put them on your skin. Then the toxins enter your bloodstream and create more detoxification work for your liver. The most efficient approach is to consider only putting creams, lotions, etc., on your skin if they are directly derived from healthy, edible products and have no added synthetic chemicals. This will simplify life and propel you forward into your new youthing lifestyle.

A. Bathing, Showering and Soaking

Here are a few simple self-help cleansing ideas. To "exercise" your blood vessels and invigorate your entire body, try incorporating a hot and cold shower regimen. On the simple end of the spectrum, you can shower with warm or hot water, and end with cool or cold. Ending with cool or cold water closes your skin's pores and redirects your blood flow to your vital organs. For a greater challenge (and more health benefit), you can alternate between several cycles of hot followed by cold water. Use thirty to sixty seconds for each hot and cold segment. In addition to improving your circulation, which promotes detoxification, you will also improve your immunity and skin texture.

Look for a filter for your shower or bathtub to neutralize or remove chloramine or chlorine at the very least. Numerous choices are available online. Several ball filters (a round ball that fits directly under the tub's spigot) are possible choices for cleaner soaking. Another method is to add 1000 mg (about one teaspoon) of vitamin C powder to your freshly drawn tub of water. Let it work on purifying your tub water for three to five minutes before you begin soaking. If you typically shower, more options are available for shower-head filters. At least one model has a cartridge of vitamin C that is slowly emitted to neutralize the chloramine, but may not be effective in neutralizing other toxins found in your tap water.

> **Vitamin C**
> Vitamin C effectively neutralizes chlorine and is safer to handle than sulfur-based dechlorination chemicals. The sodium ascorbate form of vitamin C has less effect on pH than the ascorbic acid form. When neutralizing a strong chlorine solution, both forms of vitamin C will slightly lower the dissolved oxygen of the treated water. If passive dechlorination is not practical, we recommend supplementing with a form of vitamin C.[5]

Immediately before showering or soaking in your tub, it is beneficial to use a skin brush (a long-handled natural bristle brush) to gently scrub and exfoliate your limbs, torso and neck. Brush with a circular motion, moving from the extremities—fingers and toes—toward the heart. This promotes proper circulation, takes off dead skin and surface toxins, and stimulates the pores, as well as your skin's oil glands. Skin brushing can give you a fresh clean feeling, a great way to start your day.

Detoxing baths are valuable ways to relax as you detoxify. There are several options for doing this. One of my favorites is to use approximately two cups of Epsom salts or magnesium flakes in a tub of comfortably-warm to tolerably-hot water. You can add essential oils of your choice for therapeutic benefits and fragrance. Another option is to add two or more cups of apple cider vinegar to your bath. You can experiment by using Epsom salts on one occasion and apple cider vinegar on another occasion to determine which your body finds more desirable. Both methods encourage toxins to exit through your skin's pores. Your Clinical Kinesiology self-testing skills can also help to determine whether the Epsom salts or the apple cider vinegar are the best for you. If your body is significantly more compatible with one, then by all means use the item with the strongest muscle test response.

After your bath or shower avoid using chemical-laden hygienic and cosmetic products on your skin. Instead, turn to more natural alternatives. For instance, I make my own deodorant by using one part liquid colloidal silver (available in your health food store or online), two parts filtered water, and a few drops of organic lemon essential

> **Review of Muscle-Response Testing**
>
> You may also want to refer back to the section on muscle testing in the Introduction of this book, page(s) xvii-xviii.
>
> 1. Be sure to maintain *mental neutrality* as you perform a "basic indicator muscle test" or series of tests first.
> 2. Perform the test by having a container of each substance nearby and individually testing your muscle response for each one.
> 3. Hold the first test item (like the Epsom salts) in your hand or balance it on your lap while you or your testing partner checks your body for compatibility.
> 4. Make note of the response as per muscle strength, and then test the other item or items in turn.
> 5. The item with the strongest test response should be your detoxing bath method of choice.

oil. Another very interesting deodorant that helps to detoxify (instead of compounding toxicity) is Primal Pit Paste™ (www.primalpitpaste.com). This cleansing deodorant is made from organic oils, organic butters (like Shea butter), and numerous food-grade ingredients. PiperWai is another effective and non-toxic deodorant. It contains activated charcoal as the active ingredient, but does not leave black residue. Baking soda is the only dusting power I ever use.

> **Warning on Talcum Powder**
>
> The use of talcum powder has been correlated with occurrences of ovarian cancer.[6]

More Soaking and Steaming Ideas

If you enjoy relaxing in water or swimming you may wish to add the pleasure of outdoor, natural hot-spring soaking to your regimen. I have several favorite locations in my vicinity. A search online may reveal the closest possibility for you. Go to www.soak.net for a state-by-state guide. Many hot springs have pools of different water temperatures, from comfortably warm to super-hot. These springs boast various mineral contents and some offer a mud bath, which is a great skin exfoliant and softener. Happy soaking!

You may want to check in with your doctor or natural healthcare practitioner before embarking on other detoxification methods such as using a sauna, or steam bath, or a therapeutic footbath treatment. Most commonly, saunas and steam baths are available at spas, recreation centers and athletic centers. Some people are lucky enough to have one in their home and these can be quite beneficial as they encourage your body to move toxins out through your sweat pores. You will want to be sure that your blood pressure and other health factors are at a level that qualifies you for one of these relaxing and detoxifying treatments.

I have used a therapeutic footbath treatment for myself for many years, and have also made this available to my patients We have found it to be beneficial. I prefer the Aqua Chi® instrument and have actually had my pre-treatment and post-treatment water tested by a reputable laboratory. Notable increases of numerous toxic and heavy metals were verified after my treatment. Check with your holistic health practitioner if you wish to have this treatment, as it may cleanse medications from your system more rapidly than normal. In some cases, it is advisable to do this detoxification treatment in the morning prior to taking certain medications. In other cases this may be contraindicated or unsuitable for certain individuals. This especially applies to those taking anti-rejection drugs after an organ transplant.

> ### Check First
> Many more rigorous detoxification treatments procedures and protocols are available. Consulting with a natural healthcare practitioner who can monitor your condition, your need for detoxification, as well as your progress is advisable.

B. Nontoxic Tooth and Mouth Care

Continue to incorporate non-toxic and natural measures into all aspects of your lifestyle. While it may seem simple to take care of your teeth and mouth, the potential for either increasing your body's toxic load or diminishing it rests in making educated, but simple decisions in this domain as well. I alternate between types of dental cleansers to give my body variety and to avoid building up tolerance to a certain product or formula. This same principal can be applied to skin cleanser, moisturizer and lotion choices, cosmetic choices, and even food choices. A varied diet adds a broader spectrum of nutrients, and diminishes the likelihood of developing food sensitivities.

For toothpaste, I alternate between using my own baking-soda and sea-salt mixture (sometimes adding essential oils or powdered minerals), and a natural, herbal toothpaste made by the Herbal Dental Company® that does not have toxic fluoride or sweeteners added. For more variety, I sometimes choose a probiotic toothpaste, or a clay and sea salt variety (called Earthpaste®).

> **Simple Tooth Powder**
> 1 part baking soda
> 1 part salt (select finely ground Hain® sea salt or table salt)
> Mix together

Commercial-grade toothpaste that you find in your pharmacy, grocery store, or big box store undoubtedly will have sodium fluoride (a toxic industrial byproduct that is carcinogenic), one or more types of sweeteners, and a few other chemicals thrown in. It's interesting to note that fluoride-containing toothpaste tubes display warning labels directing you to contact the poison control center if you swallow the product. **Reading labels and doing the research to understand what you've read** is a proactive, health-promoting principle that empowers you to "keep the toxins-out" of your regimen. An interesting sidenote, even some veterinarians advise against using commercial fluoride toothpaste on your pet's teeth because of the toxicity.

C. Oil Pulling

Beyond brushing your teeth, you can benefit your mouth, teeth, gums and tongue as well as your entire body by incorporating a simple detoxification method called "oil pulling." Many people believe this to be an ancient Ayurvedic health practice (*Ayurveda* is a health system from India that has existed for millennia). Oil pulling involves simply taking approximately one ounce of a healthy oil in its natural unprocessed state, such as organic, cold-pressed coconut oil, sunflower oil, or sesame oil and swishing it around in your mouth. Your goal is to avoid swallowing the oil while holding it in your mouth for ten-to-fifteen minutes and vigorously or actively swishing and/or "chewing" the oil. At the end of your fifteen minutes, or at the endpoint of your tolerance for swishing oil, whichever comes first, spit the oil out. Often I use a square of folded paper towel to catch the oil and observe the residue. The goal is to use the oil as a cleansing agent; it will osmotically draw toxins from the lining of your mouth and your tongue. You can spit the oil directly into a wastebasket or into the toilet, but it will leave a residue which will require extra cleaning. Next, you should rinse your mouth two or three times, scrape your tongue with a tongue-scraping tool (or simply a spoon) to remove residue that you may have been unaware of, and then brush your teeth. The process has a learning curve, and you have to train your tongue and lips to cooperate. It's best to stand near a wastebasket or sink during the first few attempts. Eventually, you will be able to multitask: wash your face or shave, wash a few dishes or perform other simple tasks while swishing away. I have observed my patients' teeth become whiter after they have been oil pulling several times a week for approximately six months. This is a simple and inexpensive procedure that can effectively help with detoxification. Dr. Bruce Fife's book, *Oil Pulling Therapy* (see Learn More: Books at the end of the chapter), will give you more information on this healthful practice.

D. Colon Cleansing

Like so much of the population, maturing adults in this Western culture are often plagued with inefficient bowel elimination and even outright constipation, one symptom of poor digestive health. In this section we will focus on this topic from a variety of perspectives, all leading to more effective bowel elimination and therefore more rapid toxin elimination.

Digestive Enzymes

Your body has several systems in place to help you eliminate waste and toxins. We have already discussed the skin, your largest eliminative organ. Your intestinal tract is composed of several organs that have coordinated functions. It is the second largest, and most recognized, eliminative system in your body. If your digestive system is well tuned and properly functioning, you will easily absorb beneficial nutrients from your healthy food selections and promptly and efficiently eliminate toxic-waste residue.

Research has shown that many people over the age of forty have a suboptimal level of digestive enzyme production.[7] Ensuring the presence of digestive enzymes with each meal helps you to digest your food more thoroughly and prepares the waste for elimination. Balancing your internal pH levels helps stimulate your body to ramp up production of digestive enzymes. For more information on digestive enzymes, you can refer back to pages 72 and 91 in Chapter 5. Ingesting an herbal bitters mixture five or ten minutes prior to meals may help trigger your stomach to make hydrochloric acid that boosts digestion of proteins and fats, and then trigger your pancreas to produce its specific digestive enzymes. Below is my recipe for a simple Do-It-Yourself herbal bitters formula that you can make at home to boost your digestive efficiency.

Dr. Levy's Simple Digestive Blend™ Recipe
(I make this remedy in two-ounce batches, using one ounce of each herb.)
- 1 part organic gentian herbal tincture
- 1 part organic anise herbal tincture

1. Stir the mixture thoroughly
2. Carefully pour into two one-ounce dropper bottles.

> 3. Tighten dropper caps.
> 4. Wash and dry the outsides of the bottles to remove any brown and sticky residue.
> 5. Label the bottles.
> 6. Keep one bottle on the kitchen table or in a convenient and noticeable spot.
> 7. Keep one bottle in a cup holder of your car to have available when eating away from home. (Or plan another way to have this liquid handy when dining out.)
> 8. Be careful not to expose the mixture to temperatures exceeding 100 degrees F or 37 degrees C by leaving it in your car during summer months.

For the best effect, take four-to-ten drops in a few ounces of water prior to meals. If this enzyme stimulator was forgotten prior to a meal, it can be taken afterwards.

Use your Clinical Kinesiology skills to determine your specific dosage. (Review the Clinical Kinesiology testing protocol on pages xvii-xviii.) Prior to eating your meal, do the preliminary indicator-muscle-test while sitting. Avoid looking at your plate or bowl. A testing partner can be helpful. Next, look at and smell the aroma of your meal and ask the question: "Is my body now prepared to digest this meal optimally?" If you have a weak response, proceed to test for dosage of Dr. Levy's Simple Digestive Blend™. Add four drops to a small glass of water, take a sip and repeat the question and test. If the response is weak again, increase in one drop increments and retest until a strong muscle response is attained. If you do not have a strong response with ten drops, it will be best to re-do the testing several hours later, search for an alternative product, or consult your trusted Clinical Kinesiologist.

Many other digestive enzyme formulations and products are available, and one of these may be just right for you. You can test any other digestive helpers with the same procedure. Most digestive enzyme formulations are effective in dosages of one or two tablets or capsules per meal. If you take betaine hydrochloride (often called HCl), be sure to take it three to five minutes after a meal. This allows your own acid production to occur prior to supplementing.

Fiber for Your Best Elimination
Incorporating more dietary fiber into your meals is another proactive way to keep your digestive system functioning well, and to promote effective bowel elimination.

Highest Fiber-Containing Foods[8]

Navy beans, cooked	1 cup	19 grams of fiber
Yellow beans, cooked	1 cup	18 grams of fiber
French beans, cooked	1 cup	17 grams of fiber
Peas, split, cooked	1 cup	16 grams of fiber
Pinto beans, cooked	1 cup	15 grams of fiber
Peas, green, frozen	1 cup	14 grams of fiber
Pinion nuts	1 ounce	12 grams of fiber
Oat bran, raw	½ cup	12 grams of fiber
Acorn squash	1 cup	9 grams of fiber
Avocado, raw	½ fruit	9 grams of fiber
Figs, dried	½ cup	8 grams of fiber
Pear	1 medium	6 grams of fiber

In studying African tribal people who foraged and hunted for their food, Dr. Denis Parsons Burkitt, M.D. found that these people typically had a one-to-one ratio of bowel movements to meals per day. In other words, one bowel movement per day is normal if **only** one meal is consumed. I was fortunate enough to attend one of Dr. Burkitt's lectures and meet him in person. Two of his graphics for the presentation were highly illustrative, and epitomized his entire lecture.

The first slide demonstrated an African tribal person squatting to defecate in the jungle, leaving behind a large "pile." In the background was a sketch of a small rudimentary clinic. The second slide depicted an urban person sitting on a toilet seat struggling to eject small, hard "nuggets." Dr. Burkitt sketched a large medical center complex in the background of his drawing. He writes:

> *America is a constipated nation...If you pass small stools, you have to have large hospitals...Western diets are so low on bulk and so dense in calories, that our intestines just don't pass enough volume to remain healthy.*[9]

Avoiding processed foods, especially flour-based foods, is the key to a high-fiber diet for most people. Including a high percentage of plant-based foods is the next step. Some find it helpful to add a fiber supplement. Squatting, or elevating your feet on a telephone book or other prop at least six-inches high, reduces the strain on your intestinal tract and facilitates the bowel movement. The Squatty Potty® is a seven-inch-high footstool to use while on your toilet. You can learn more information about this product at squattypotty.com.

Guidance in Choosing a Fiber Supplement
- No added sugar or artificial sweeteners
- No added flavorings
- No added colorants
- Choose a balance of soluble and insoluble fiber. (They occur together in unprocessed foods.)
- Ground seeds are often used: Flaxseed, chia seeds and psyllium
- Apple pectin, acacia gum powder, oat bran and inulin (a prebiotic) are also common in the higher quality fiber products.

I recommend Organic Triple Fiber from Renew Life® and Favao™ fiber made by Xango® as two easily accessed products. I frequently recommend specific fiber formulations made by nutrient companies that serve natural healthcare providers. Your Clinical Kinesiologist or natural healthcare practitioner can help you with professional-grade fiber formulations. You or your healthcare practitioner can use Clinical

Kinesiology to test two or more fiber products to determine which one gives you the strongest muscle test response.

Caution: Always stir your powdered fiber supplement into at least eight ounces of water (add one or two ounces of juice for flavor if you need to for palatability) and immediately drink it prior to it thickening. Following this up with additional water is advisable. If your fiber supplement is in capsule or tablet form, you also need to take it with eight-to-twelve ounces of water so that it expands and goes to work in your intestinal tract. When fiber supplements are taken with an insufficient amount of water, they may thicken and harden. This may contribute to constipation by further slowing the elimination process.

Enemas

If you have not been regularly having one large, soft-formed bowel movement per meal each day, you are probably harboring a surprising amount of waste in the crevices and curves of your large intestine. High-fiber foods, digestive enzymes and fiber supplements may help your situation, but you may also benefit from an enema. Enemas may deliver relief to someone who is acutely constipated and may even help wash out and dilute stubborn waste material that has collected on the colon walls over time.

> **Enema Warning**
>
> Only proceed with doing your own enema after you have determined that you do not have a health condition that makes this treatment inadvisable. Extreme constipation that has caused a fecalith (or fecal stone), uncontrolled coronary heart disease, rectal prolapse, previous colon surgery, colon cancer, chemotherapy and colitis are examples of conditions that can contraindicate self-administered enemas.[10] If you do not have a concern about doing your own enema, research the procedure and become fully acquainted with the protocol and its nuances before performing this procedure.

Generally, an enema involves the use of an enema bag and approximately one quart of comfortably warm water. Most people lie on their left side on a towel or rug near the toilet. This allows the water to flow into the sigmoid and descending colon. By increments, slowly release a few ounces of water into the rectum and close the clamp on your tubing. Attempt to hold this water for three-to-five minutes. When you experience a strong urge to release, get up and release the water and waste material in the toilet. As you are more accustomed to the process you will be able to hold more and more ounces of water before releasing.

A colonic or colon hydrotherapy treatment is administered by a trained colon therapist and uses a therapeutic colonic irrigation device to gradually and intermittently deliver up to several gallons of water, interspersed with ample time to release waste and water, prior to the next fill cycle. The same list of contraindications that applied to enemas also applies to colon hydrotherapy.

Your classically trained medical doctor may be unfamiliar with or fearful of this treatment, but the majority of natural healthcare practitioners will be knowledgeable about this valuable therapeutic and cleansing methodology. Educate yourself about colon hydrotherapy by looking at the website for The International Association for Colon Hydrotherapy at www.I-ACT.org. Meet with a therapist that you are considering working with for more education, and to view the equipment and facility, before committing to a session.

I encourage you to continue your research about colon cleansing. Educational materials on this topic are abundant.

E. Cosmetic Detox, More Than Just A Pretty Face

If there are forty-two different cosmetic and bodycare items in your bathroom, you could potentially be harboring and using several hundred human-made chemicals. Reading about some of these ingredients can be frightening. One example is that red lipstick frequently contains lead, arsenic and/or cadmium. Yes, these are some of nature's elements, but they can be quite harmful. In fact, upon testing, one of these lip glosses contained 110 ppm of lead which was ten times over the allowable limit by the guidelines of the Canadian agency that regulates cosmetics. Even though no cases of toxic or heavy-metal poisoning are documented stemming from this lipstick, it certainly seems prudent to either avoid lipstick or avoid using those with heavy metals as a component.

Other cosmetics, including skin cleansers, lotion, shampoos, hair conditioners and the like contain a variety of synthetically-made chemicals responsible for shocking, deleterious effects, including cancer. For those who choose to use makeup, there are varieties of mineral makeup, free of lead, arsenic and cadmium available. For a shampoo, I prefer Juni™, natural shampoo and conditioner made by Xango®. They leave my hair soft and shiny. Juni™ also provides a pure skin lotion.

Another way to reduce or eliminate toxic cosmetics is to use organic natural oil on your skin instead of lotion. I use Egyptian Magic® on my face and hands frequently. Egyptian magic is made of olive oil, honey and bee pollen. Most commercially available skin lotions and cosmetics contain phthalates, paraben preservatives, formaldehyde derivatives and other toxic agents that are known carcinogens.[11] Check out the websites Wellness Mama (www.wellnessmama.com) and Our Nourishing Roots (www.ournourishingroots.com) to learn about making your own cosmetics with simple natural ingredients. And/or, you can visit your local healthfood store and ask about high quality all-natural health and body care products. Two of my favorite companies for facial skincare are Glimpse™ by Xango®, and Lily Organics®, an organic, farm-based cottage industry. Both use all-natural ingredients and avoid synthetic chemicals.

Another of your "keep the toxins out" principles could be: **"Simple and clean; no artificial chemicals for me!"**

F. Detox Through Sleep And Rest

We have all probably experienced the negative side effects of sleep deficiency.[12] Sleep and adequate rest are necessary for everyone at any age, but it can be especially important for elders. Your body (especially your liver and brain) uses the "down time" while you sleep to detoxify itself. Research shows that the glymphatic system, the part of your central nervous system that helps eliminate waste "ramps up its activity during sleep, thereby allowing your brain to clear out toxins, including harmful proteins linked to brain disorders such as Alzheimer's for example. What's more, they discovered that your brain cells actually shrink by about 60 percent during sleep, which allows for more efficient waste removal."[13]

Poor-quality or an insufficient quantity of sleep can also "contribute to premature aging by interfering with your growth hormone production, normally released by your pituitary gland during deep sleep."[14]

You may choose to keep a diary or a simple log, even make notations on your calendar concerning the amount of downtime or relaxation and actual sleep that you get. Correlate your rest and sleep with your vibrancy and high-energy days on paper so that you may clearly appreciate the correlation between the two. If you can see the connection between your lower functioning days and your sleep deficiency days the recording project will prove worthwhile.

Good sleep hygiene starts with a sensible and consistent bedtime and waking time…If you have a flood of thoughts running through your mind when you go to bed, you can train your mind to do a "data dump" before going to the bedroom… A logical consideration is to search for a mind-body issue, a trapped emotion, or an unexpressed need. This type of issue may be difficult to identify. Once it is identified and addressed, stress and sleep difficulties may improve or abate.[15]

SIMPLE DO-IT-YOURSELF DETOX HELPERS

Liver

Herbs	Foods and Freshly Made Juices	Other Measures
Artichoke leaf	Artichoke	Castor oil pack put onto skin topically
Cayenne Milk thistle	Avocado	Chlorella pills, powder, or liquid as a supplement
Dandelion root and leaves	Beets	Cleansing clay as a supplement (1 teaspoon powder stirred into water; drink daily or as directed by healthcare professional
Fennel	Cauliflower	
Ginger	Fresh dandelion leaves	
	Garlic	
	Leafy greens	
	Lemon	
	Milk thistle seeds	

The Liver Flush[16]
1 orange
½ grapefruit
½ lemon
6-8 oz. of water
2-4-6 oz. pure olive oil (gradually increase daily)
2 tablespoons cut raw ginger root or garlic
Process all ingredients in a blender and drink in the morning. Wait two or three hours before eating food.

Kidney

Herbs	Foods and Freshly Made Juices	Other Measures
Artichoke leaf	Artichoke	Drink Pure water
Dandelion root and leaves	Asparagus	Spirulina pills or powder as a supplement
Ginger	Carrot	
Goldenrod	Celery	
Horsetail	Cranberry	
Parsley	Cucumber	
Stinging nettles	Grapes	
	Purple cabbage	
	Radish	
	Spinach	
	String beans	
	Watered down lime juice	
	Watermelon	

Lymphatic System

Herbs	Food and Freshly Made Juices	Other Measures
Astragalus	Lemon	Activated charcoal capsules (black stools are normal after consumption)
Burdock		Lymphatic massages
Cayenne		Mini-trampoline (jump three to five minutes and increase duration as tolerated)
Chaparral		Pure water

Herbs	Food and Freshly Made Juices	Other Measures
Cleavers		Skin brushing
Parsley		
Poke root		
Red clover		
Stillingia		

Whole Body

Other Measures	Food and Freshly Made Juices	Other Measures
Cilantro	Apples	Activated charcoal capsules (black stools are normal after consumption)
Ginger	Avocado	Chlorella pills or powder as a supplement
Parsley	Beets	Cleansing clay as a supplement (1 teaspoon powder stirred into water; drink daily or as directed by healthcare professional)
	Cabbage (all types)	Massage
	Celery	Pure water
	Garlic	Skin brushing
	Kale	Zeolite mineral powder as a supplement (1 teaspoon stirred into water; drink daily or as directed by healthcare professional)
	Pears	
	Seaweed	

CONCLUSION

I suggest rereading and referring back to this Detox chapter often because it can serve as a basic guide to your understanding of how to keep the toxins out of your body. Everything in this chapter can support your health and longevity-building strategies.

Toxic residues of your normal body metabolism, as well as nefarious chemical toxins from your environment and previous dietary choices lay the foundation for inflammatory processes. This vital topic of inflammation will be examined in the next chapter.

LEARN MORE
- To read more about the vitally important bacteria in your intestinal tract read pages 156-160 in *Your Body Can Talk, 2nd Edition*
- To read more about liver detoxification and the Liver Flush procedure, read pages 193-194 in *Your Body Can Talk, 2nd Edition*
- To read more about good sleep hygiene read pages 336-341 in *Your Body Can Talk, 2nd Edition*

Books
Fife, Bruce, N.D. *Oil Pulling Therapy: Detoxifying and Healing the Body Through Oral Cleansing.* Colorado Springs, Colo.: Piccadilly Books, Ltd., 2008.

Flanagan, Deuce. *Everybody Poops 410 Pounds a Year: An Illustrated Bathroom Companion for Grown-Ups.* Berkeley, Calif.: Ulysses Press, 2010.

Malkan, Stacy. *Not Just a Pretty Face: The Ugly Side of the Beauty Industry.* Gabriola Island, BC, Canada: New Society Publishers, 2007.

Morse, Robert, S., N.D. *The Detox Miracle Sourcebook: Raw Foods and Herbs for Complete Cellular Regeneration.* Prescott, Ariz.: Kalindi Press, 2004.

Smith, Jeffery. *Genetic Roulette: The Documented Health Risks of Genetically Engineered Foods, 4th Edition.* Fairfield, Iowa: Yes! Books, 2007.

Websites
A state-by-state guide for natural hot springs: www.soak.net
Our Nourishing Roots: www.ournourishing roots.com

The International Association for Colon Hydrotherapy: www.I-ACT.org

Wellness Mama: www.wellnessmama.com

Products

Aqua Chi® Foot Baths: http://www.aquachifootbath.com/

Berkey® Water purification and filtration system: http://www.berkeyfilters.com/

CedarCide® Safe, Organic Bug Control: https://www.cedarcide.com/

Dr. Bronner's Liquid Soap Cleaning Agent: https://www.drbronner.com/DBMS/category/LIQUIDSOAP.html

Earthpaste® Clay and Sea-Salt Based Toothpaste: http://www.earthpaste.com/

Egyptian Magic® Skin Cream: http://naturallikeus.com

Favao™ fiber by Xango®: http://mymangosteen.com/DrSusan/product/favao_fiber.asp

Glimpse Mineral Makeup: http://mymangosteen.com/DrSusan/product/mineral_treatment.asp

Glimpse™ facial skin care products by Xango®: http://mymangosteen.com/DrSusan/product/glimpse.asp

Gonzo Odor Eliminator™ Volcanic Rock Odor Eliminator: https://gonzoproducts.com/All-Products/Odor-Eliminator

Herbal Dental Company® Fluoride and Sweetener Free Tooth Care Products: https://www.dentalherb.com/

Juni™ natural shampoo, conditioner and skin lotion by Xango®: http://mymangosteen.com/DrSusan/product/juni.asp

Lily Organics® Organic Facial Skin Care Products: https://lilyfarmfreshskincare.com/

Multipure® Water Purification and Filtration System: http://www.multipure.com/

Molly's Suds Non-Toxic Laundry Soap: https://mollyssuds.com/products/

Organic Triple Fiber from Renew Life®: http://www.renewlife.com/fiber-supplements/triple-fiber-capsules.html

PiperWai Non-Toxic, Charcoal Based Deodorant: https://www.piperwai.com/

Primal Pit Paste™: Cleansing Deodorant Made from Organic Oils, Organic Butters, and Numerous Food-Grade Ingredients: http://primalpitpaste.com/
Squatty Potty® Ergonomic Foot Stool: http://www.squattypotty.com/
The MoSo Bags® Bamboo Charcoal Odor Eliminator: http://www.mosonatural.com/
Zeolite Mineral Powder: https://www.zeolite.com/
ZEROREZ® Water Based Carpet Cleaner: http://www.zerorez.com/

Endnotes, Chapter 6

1. Claudio, Luz. Planting Healthier Indoor Air. *Environmental Health Perspectives*, 119, no. 10 (2011). Accessed March 20, 2016. (http://www.ncbi.nlm.nih.gov/pmc/articles/PMC3230460/)
2. Wolverton, B.C. Ph.D., Anne Johnson, M.S. and Keith Bounds, M.S. Interior Landscape Plants for Indoor Air Pollution Abatement. *NASA Office of Commercial Programs—Technology Utilization Division, and the Associated Landscape Contractors of America (ALCA)*. Sept. 15, 1989. Accessed March 20, 2016 (http://ntrs.nasa.gov/archive/nasa/casi.ntrs.nasa.gov/19930073077.pdf)
3. MoSo Natural. "What is a Moso Bag." Moso Natural, 2016. Accessed March 20, 2106, http://www.moso natural.com/what-is-a-moso-bag/
4. Berman, Marc G., John Jonides and Stephen Kaplan. "The Cognitive Benefits of Interacting with Nature." *Psychological Science*. 19:12 (2008): 1207-1212. https://pdfs.semanticscholar.org/5cef/86418e03740fc1a77eff6ba0b10541a2e223.pdf (accessed March 22, 2016).
5. Land, Brenda. "Using Vitamin C to Neutralize Chlorine in Water Systems." *United States Department of Agriculture Forest Services, Technology and Development Program: Recreation Management Tech Tips*, April 2005. Accessed April 20, 2016. http://www.fs.fed.us/t-d/pubs/html/05231301/05231301.html
6. "Talcum Powder and Ovarian Cancer." *Drug Watch* March 9, 2016. (accessed March 22, 2016). https://www.drugwatch.com/talcum-powder/ovarian-cancer/
7. "Digestive Disorders: Steps to a Healthier Digestive System." *Life Extension: Health Concerns*. 2016. Accessed April 20, 2016. http://www.lifeextension.com/protocols/gastrointestinal/digestive-disorders/page-04
8. Palmer, Sharon, RD. "The Top Fiber-Rich Foods List." *Today's Dietitian*, 10, no. 7 (July 2008): 28. Accessed April 20, 2016. http://www.todaysdietitian.com/newarchives/063008p28.shtml
9. *Famous quotes by Denis Burkitt, M.D.* "The Mcdougall Newsletter: It's the Food." Accessed April 26, 2016: https://www.drmcdougall.com/misc/2013nl/jan/burkitt.htm.

10 Niv, Galia and Tamar Grinberg, Ram Dickman, Nir Wasserberg and Yaron Niv. "Perforation and Mortality After Cleansing Enema for Acute Constipation Are Not Rare but Are Preventable." *International Journal of General Medicine*. 6 (2013): 323-328.
11 Malkan, Stacy. *Not Just a Pretty Face: The Ugly Side of the Beauty Industry*. Gabriola Island, British Columbia: New Society Publishers, 2007.
12 Cedernaes, Jonathan and Megan E. Osler, Sarah Voisin, Jan-Eric Broman, Heike Vogel, Suzanne L. Dickson, Juleen R. Zierath, Helgi B. Schiöth, and Christian Benedict. "Acute Sleep Loss Induces Tissue-Specific Epigenetic and Transcriptional Alterations to Circadian Clock Genes in Men." *The Journal of Clinical Endocriology and Metabolism*. 100:9 (2015). Accessed May 5, 2016. *http://press. endocrine. org/doi/full/10.1210/JC.2015-2284*
13 "Sleep Is Critical for Brain Detoxification, Groundbreaking Research Finds." Mercola.com. Last modified October 31, 2013. http://articles.mercola.com/sites/articles/archive/2013/10/31/sleep-brain-detoxification.aspx
14 Idem.
15 Levy, 339.
16 Ibid.,193-194.

CHAPTER 7

Inflammation: The Anti-Youthing Agent

One of the first lessons an infant begins to learn is to distinguish his or her own body as something separate from others, as well as from their immediate environment. This early developmental process initiates a lifelong endeavor. Who am I? Where do I start, where do I stop? What is self? We all experience this self-discernment process from various vantage points as we move through life's phases, even into elderhood. I encourage you to continue your philosophical, spiritual and environmental quest to discern among all aspects of life what is compatible to your body and your being, and to include in your life that which is nourishing—spiritually, biologically and emotionally. In this chapter we will be considering what happens when irritating "non-self" particles, chemicals and organisms invade or come in close proximity to your body. The result is known as inflammation, and is a primary agent in premature aging and disease.

WHAT IS INFLAMMATION, AND WHY ALL THE FUSS?
Inflammation is a normal and protective immune-system reaction of your body when it is distressed, from mildly to seriously. When an oyster takes on a grain of sand or some other foreign particle, irritation builds and inflammation begins. The oyster attempts to lessen the irritation by adding layer after layer of a soothing substance it creates. The end result is a smooth pearl. Now there are no rough edges to traumatize

the soft tissues of the oyster. Your own body has numerous complicated methods of coping with and adapting to irritants as well.

For our purposes, inflammation is defined as a natural yet complex biochemical and immune response to injury, infection or toxicity. The classic signs of inflammation have been known since the time of the ancient Romans. Aulus Cornelius Celsus (25 BCE–50 CE) is credited with observing and defining the four principal signs of inflammation:

- Redness (*rubor*)
- Heat (*calor*)
- Swelling (*tumor*)
- Pain (*dolor*)

Throughout your life, the components of your immune system busy themselves with the task of identifying your own cells, tissues, body fluids, beneficial biochemicals and even beneficial bacteria. Similar components of your immune system are on an endless quest to find, segregate, capture and hopefully destroy non-self chemical and biological factors. Inside your body, functioning day-in and day-out, are built-in biochemical and cellular mechanisms intended to protect you from toxic, pathological (bacterial, viral, fungal and parasitic) invaders and otherwise harmful non-self entities. For now, we will consider these protective biochemical and cellular factors to be your personal "security guards." If you eat a life-supportive diet and follow the principles, "Eat What You Are Made of… And Trash the Rest," covered in Chapters 5 and 6, and diminish your exposure to toxins overall, you will save your protective "security guards" hours of needless work. This will increase your immunity and decrease your likelihood of chronic inflammation. Chronic inflammation is an age-accelerant because it constantly overworks your immune system; as such, it is a counter-productive agent to your youthing process.

A Brief Primer About Inflammation and Health

Your "security guards" are the active players in your immune system. Some of the most famous are your T-helper cells. These are specialized white blood cells that form in your thymus gland located just under your sternum or breastbone. T-helper cells are able to secrete biologically-active substances that have many important functions.

> **Stimulate Your Immunity**
> Gently tapping with your fingertips over your sternum for up to two-to-three minutes at a time is one way to gently stimulate your immune system and bolster your immunity. It is one simple tool you can use to help cope with inflammation.

Your T-cells and other important cells in your immune system secrete a variety of messaging substances. For our purposes, we will discuss only one group of these substances, the *cytokines*, of which there are many varieties. This modern term derives from the Greek words meaning "cell" and "movement." Cytokines are small protein molecules that are preprogrammed to seek receptor sites on specific cells and deliver them a work directive. One job your diligent cytokines perform is to direct certain white blood cells to particular locations under specific conditions. Your busy cytokines even provide a roadmap for your white blood cells. A chemical trail is laid down from point A to point B for your defender white blood cells to follow. Each time your body encounters an inflammatory trigger, relevant cytokines and other immune factors are called into action.

> **Natural or Manufactured?**
> Replicas of some cytokines have been produced using DNA technology by pharmaceutical companies. You have likely heard the name of at least one of them, Interferon®. For our purposes we are only discussing the naturally-occurring cytokines that your body makes.

Without a life-supportive diet and care in monitoring toxic intake, human beings are filling their bodies with countless toxic and biologically-purposeless packets of non-self garbage. Since these items are certainly **not** self and cannot be recognized as such, many of them will be classified as *antigens*. You can think of an antigen as a problematic chemical or organism that is immediately considered a criminal suspect in your body and will soon be surrounded on all sides by your antibodies and your "security guards": various white blood cells and natural immunity mediators. You can easily imagine the crowd that gathers when someone indulges in eating a gooey, sticky doughnut—it calls up the forces by the thousands! At some point, crowd control measures need to be undertaken—sort of like disseminating "pepper-spray" upon an unruly crowd. When that happens, the inflammatory process is in full swing.

Acute inflammation will demonstrate at least one inflammation sign (redness, heat, swelling and/or pain) soon after the injury or other precipitating stimulus. Your body's inflammatory reaction contributes to the formation of these observable signs. Any time you experience one or more of these indicators, consider that some degree of inflammation is present in your body.

If you have chronic inflammation, or toxic inflammation, these four cardinal signs are definitely at play, yet may not be as immediately observable as in acute inflammation. Sometimes the long term effects are only observed after weeks, months or years.

To explain this more graphically, think about the goldfish metaphor from Chapter 6. Imagine our goldfish in its small aquarium, and further imagine that no water change or tank cleaning has occurred for over a week. Suppose that a photo of the aquarium was taken each day during that period. As you can guess, in looking at these pictures afterward, it would be fairly obvious that any worsening of the goldfish's conditions might directly correlate to the increased murkiness of the water. The same is true for you. As toxic chemicals and biological waste progressively builds up in your tissues, your degree of inflammation will also increase. As the lives of goldfish living in murky waters are shortened, so are the lifespans of chemically-inflamed humans.

Another way to visualize toxic inflammation is to consider the example of walking or hiking with gritty sand in your shoes. The first several steps may not be very irritating, but the farther you walk with the sand rubbing the soles of your feet, the more uncomfortable, irritated and inflamed your feet become. The only reasonable solution is to stop, remove the toxin (the gritty sand) from your shoes, and then rest and pamper your feet.

Inflammation Triggers
The inflammatory response inherent in your own body is a protective mechanism. It may be called into play by a variety of triggers. Injuries resulting from blunt or sharp trauma, such as hitting your knee on the table or cutting your finger while slicing carrots, are examples of acute injuries that typically produce acute (short-term) inflammation. If you endured a significant wound or laceration, you may require wound cleaning or debridement and/or stitching (suturing). In those cases, the wounded area is slightly reinjured during treatment and this will trigger a new cycle of localized acute inflammation. Generally, acute inflammation of this sort has great potential to resolve fairly easily and expediently. That potential is affected by the person's level of health, nutrition, hydration and attentiveness to their wound. If those factors are considerably less than optimal, however, or if the injured person has an underlying chronic source of inflammation, such as diabetes, lupus, rheumatoid arthritis or another autoimmune disease, their wound-healing time may be significantly prolonged.

Velocity trauma—such as a car crash, sports injury, slipping and falling on icy concrete—or another form of direct trauma also causes an inflammatory response. The micro-tearing of muscle and/or ligament tissue causes leakage of cellular debris and tissue fluids into the muscles that produces inflammation that may continue for weeks or months, and even longer. This process can progress until it is considered chronic (long-term) inflammation. You can effectively treat velocity trauma by specifically addressing the injured tissues with ice, therapeutic ultrasound, herbal liniment, soft (low level) laser therapy, massage (geared to the level of injury and patient tolerance), chiropractic care, acupuncture and muscle and joint rehab. These methods are much more helpful than palliative anti-inflammatory or pain medication.

Medication options actually offer no treatment of the cause, which is that cellular and metabolic debris are interspersed within the damaged soft tissues. They are classified as antigenic toxins by the immune system.

Inflammation is also an inherent factor in any infection. It is a distinct process that may continue even after the infection is healed. This will depend on the severity and type of the infection, the level of health and wellness and nutritional status of the individual. Background illnesses, particularly those of an inflammatory nature such as diabetes or lupus, could extend either the infection or the inflammation, or both.

Since there are no patentable pharmaceuticals available to assist someone with toxic inflammation, very little research is available concerning how your own *toxic load* (the amount of retained toxins in your body from your diet, environment and other lifestyle factors) contributes to chronic inflammation. Learning about how your body responds to various antigens (inflammation triggers) and what the consequences of long-term inflammation can be will augment your health, your comfort and maybe even your longevity. The next step is to find ways to reduce the level of toxins coming into your body; then to proactively coax toxins out of your system. Review Chapters 5 and 6 for workable ideas.

Leaky Gut Syndrome: A Common Inflammatory Condition
Besides accidents, wounds and traumas to your system, many of which are not preventable, dietary and lifestyle choices, as well as exposure to environmental pollution can contribute to your inflammatory process. Some of these choices result in what is graphically termed "Leaky gut syndrome." This condition, which can be quite debilitating, is a less discernible route for inflammation to insidiously creep into your system.

Leaky gut syndrome infers dysfunction of the lining or mucosal membrane of the small intestine. This leakage allows problematic substances to seep from the processing areas of the small intestine prematurely into the bloodstream. In order to better understand this, envision the screen door in your home. Properly working screen doors allow fresh air, sunlight and the pleasant fragrances of nature into your home while screening out unwanted insects and debris. Let's now imagine that the screen door is damaged and has several gaping holes. Mosquitoes, flies, grasshoppers and anything blowing in the wind will blow into your home. By the same token, if your intestinal lining is damaged enough to be "leaky," all sorts of unwanted debris and "bugs" can travel right into your bloodstream.

Most problematic health conditions and disorders are various manifestations of inflammation and a state of significant imbalance of the body. Refer to the chart on pages 144 and 145 titled "Symptoms and Conditions Related to Leaky Gut Syndrome." Here you will note over seventy-eight specific inflammatory health conditions. Even some cancer researchers have concluded that chronic inflammation potentiates a host of various cancers.[1]

Consequences of Longterm or Whole-Body Inflammation?
Inflammation is both a qualifying and a precipitating factor for most disease processes. A simple rule of thumb is that practically any health condition whose last syllable is -*itis* is a "card-carrying" inflammatory disease process. Familiar examples include arthritis, bursitis, sinusitis, thyroiditis, nephritis, pancreatitis, appendicitis, dermatitis, tonsillitis and colitis. These terms describe inflammation focalized on a particular body organ or tissue. Gout is another inflammatory disorder. Other inflammatory health conditions that you may be familiar with are asthma, seasonal allergies, hay fever, and chronic bronchitis. These respiratory conditions are very much affected by food allergens and airborne allergens. It is obvious that anyone with these conditions who also indulges in cigarette smoking or other tobacco use is actually worsening their condition. It is also true that tobacco use contributes to any type of inflammatory condition.

Diabetes is known to be inflammatory in nature and is a notorious age-accelerating disorder. Other diagnostic entities that are inflammation driven include the "opathies." You may know someone with peripheral neur**opathy** (nerve inflammation) or one of the various my**opathies** (varieties of muscle inflammation disorders). Generally speaking, anyone diagnosed with one of those disorders likely has other

Symptoms and Conditions Related to Leaky Gut Syndrome[2]

Gastro-Intestinal
- Bloating
- Flatulence
- Constipation
- Diarrhea
- Liver dysfunction
- Gluten intolerance
- Food sensitivities
- Malabsorption of nutrients
- Irritable bowel syndrome
- Inflammatory bowel disease
- Crohn's disease
- Ulcerative colitis
- Abdominal discomfort

Nervous System, Brain and Mind
- Autism
- (Apparent) Hyperactivity
- Multiple sclerosis
- Confusion
- Mental fogginess
- Poor memory
- Mood swings
- Depression
- Headaches
- Migraines
- Anxiety
- Insomnia
- Schizophrenia

Inflammation
- Swelling—muscles, face, hands, feet, joints, soft tissues, etc.
- Intestinal tract inflammation
- Fibromyalgia
- Organ dysfunction—liver, thyroid, heart pancreas, etc.

Total Body or General Symptoms
- Chronic fatigue
- Constant hunger
- Weight gain
- Difficult weight loss
- Insomnia
- Accelerated aging
- Body or joint aches and pains
- Fibromyalgia
- Multiple chemical sensitivities
- Sensitive to weather changes
- Arthritis
- Malnutrition
- Hormonal disruption (i.e., worsening of PMS, menopause, andropause, etc.)

Respiratory System
- Asthma
- Cystic fibrosis
- Nasal congestion
- Sinus issues
- Chronic sinus infection
- Shortness of breath

Symptoms and Conditions Related to Leaky Gut Syndrome[2]

Skin Issues
- Flushing—especially of face
- Acne
- Dermatitis
- Eczema
- Psoriasis
- Rashes
- Itching
- Hives
- Rosacea
- Hair loss

Decreased Immune Function
- Repeated bouts of colds, flu, sore throats, abscessing teeth, candida
- Fevers of unknown origin
- Food sensitivities and allergies
- Environmental sensitivities and allergies

Autoimmune Disorders***
- Systemic lupus erythematosus
- Chronic fatigue syndrome
- Hypothyroidism
- Hashimoto's thyroiditis
- Multiple sclerosis
- Inflammatory bowel syndrome
- Ulcerative colitis
- Crohn's disease
- Asthma
- Diabetes type II
- Rheumatoid arthritis
- Fibromyalgia
- Reiter's syndrome

***A chronic state of inflammation and immune dysfunction may evolve into an autoimmune disorder.

inflammatory processes in their body as well. It is safe to assume that all auto-immune disorders are also inflammatory disorders.

Can Inflammation Affect Brain Function?

Several mental health conditions are also associated with inflammation. Some of these include confusion, mental fogginess, mood swings and dementia. Inflammation is also related to anxiety, depression, insomnia and schizophrenia. During my days working as a registered nurse, I assisted in a private psychiatric hospital for several months. There I observed a clear relationship between the consumption of sugar, sweets, sodas and "junk food" and subsequent behavioral outbursts and extreme episodes termed as "acting out." Unfortunately, such "treats" are used as rewards for good behavior, yet ironically precipitate negative or dangerous behavior within an hour after consumption.

> ### Ruth's Story
> One of my patients, whom we will call Ruth, came to my office suffering from intractable asthma. She was fifty-seven years old. Ruth had been a premature baby whose mother was a heavy smoker and did not stop smoking during her pregnancies. Ruth was diagnosed with asthma at the age of two after numerous visits to the hospital. She had resigned herself to the thought that she would always be an asthmatic, always require various inhalers and medications, and never be physically active.
>
> During her intake exam she explained that she was an accountant for a large corporation. Each day for lunch she ate what she considered to be a seemingly simple and light meal, direct from the company cafeteria. These lunches consisted of processed ham or lunchmeat, white sandwich bread, mayonnaise and a sparse amount of iceberg lettuce with a slice of something that resembled a tomato. Ruth also enjoyed the accompanying bag of potato chips each day. She washed this all down with a can of diet soda and only treated herself to a brownie two or three days a week. At home her meals were also far from exemplary.
>
> Ruth knew she had to change something because her medications were no longer keeping her airways comfortably open. She was amazed to learn that her diet was largely pro-inflammatory and was progressively worsening her condition, but was excited about the prospect of finding a way to truly improve her asthmatic condition. She committed herself to a nutritious and toxin-free diet and vowed never again to purchase the cafeteria food.
>
> Ruth opened the door to the wide world of healthy natural foods and a largely plant-based diet. She was a star patient and proactively revamped her lifestyle. She came to weekly sessions for

> Clinical-Kinesiology-guided acupuncture and chiropractic care, and faithfully adhered to a regimen of inflammation-reducing and lung-supportive nutrients. After three months she felt a significant improvement in her health and we diminished her treatment program accordingly. By seven months after beginning treatment, Ruth felt no inclination to use her inhalers and laid them aside. Within nine months after looking for a new path, Ruth joined a hiking club and participated in progressively more challenging hikes at higher and higher elevations. By that time she only came to my office about three or four times a year for a touchup treatment and told me that she knew in her heart that she no longer had asthma.

How Do I Know if I Have Problematic Inflammation?

First, you should refer back to the definition of inflammation. You can exclude recent bumps and bruises, cuts and nicks, and ask yourself whether you are experiencing localized or generalized redness, hot-to-the-touch areas, swelling or pain. YES to any of these correlates to some unknown degree of inflammation.

The more important question is, "Is it problematic?" If you are experiencing one or more of the cardinal signs of inflammation (pain, swelling, heat, redness) frequently or consistently, that would qualify as problematic. If you are not able to identify any one of these cardinal signs, yet have been diagnosed with an inflammatory disorder or do not feel your best, you should set out to find help evaluating yourself for problematic inflammation with your trusted healthcare provider. A simple laboratory test that identifies generalized inflammation is the **C-reactive protein test**. This may be a helpful tool in some cases, but should not be the only determining factor. Checking in with your holistic healthcare practitioner and/or your primary healthcare provider and discussing your concerns is a reasonable approach.

In addition to those steps, you can test yourself with Clinical Kinesiology. Dr. Alan Beardall discovered the inflammation finger mode that Clinical Kinesiology practitioners still use today. To do this, sit comfortably in your chair to do a preliminary test on your indicator muscle to be sure you are ready for testing. Then, test the indicator muscle with your other hand. If the muscle is strong you can continue.

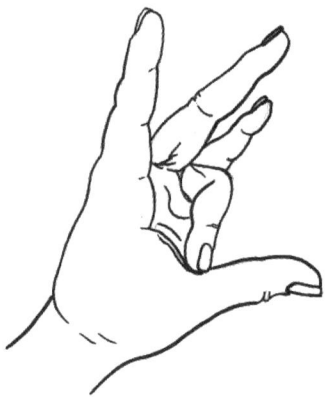

Now, you are ready to perform the inflammation finger mode. Begin by bending your fourth or "ring" finger down to the crease at the beginning of your fleshy thumb pad, making firm contact. The fingerprint of your fourth finger should be touching the crease where the thumb attaches to the palm. The next step is to hold the inflammation finger mode as you repeat the indicator muscle test. If your muscle response is weak while holding the finger mode, this indicates a great likelihood of inflammation being present. Check in with your Clinical Kinesiologist or healthcare practitioner for deeper evaluation.

If you are working with a professional, your Clinical Kinesiology practitioner will be able to specifically test various areas of the body, or tissues or organs, for the presence of inflammation. Your Clinical Kinesiology practitioner will also be able to evaluate the impact of foods, beverages, herbs and supplements on the inflammation. This might be the perfect time for you to undergo food sensitivity testing with your Clinical Kinesiology practitioner.

How Can I Help Myself Reduce Inflammation?
It is critically important to eliminate "fiery" or inflammatory agents from your lifestyle. For instance, consider that whiskey was called "firewater" in the not-too-distant past. Alcoholic beverages act as

solvents in your system. The essential fatty acids anywhere in your body are likely to be broken down by alcohol. Since most people are proportionally deficient in the omega 3 anti-inflammatory essential fatty acids, it seems counterproductive to dissolve away any portion of that precious commodity. Alcoholic beverages can also diminish or inactivate any of your fat-soluble vitamins. The delicate protective coverings of your brain and all of your nerves are also vulnerable to the solvent activity of "firewater." Anyone suffering from problematic inflammation is advised that consuming alcohol is not beneficial.

Cigarette smoking and tobacco use wreak significant havoc on your body as well. If you watch a burning cigarette you will notice that the essence of the cigarette is consumed by fire that requires extra oxygen for that process. If you puff on that burning cigarette, understand that it will be taking oxygen away from all of your tissues while leaving behind a smoky, toxic residue. Every square inch of your body requires a sufficient supply of oxygen to properly function. Smoking belongs on your Trash-It list.

Another way to defend against problematic inflammation is to allow yourself sufficient rest and sleep. During sleep your body automatically works on detoxifying, rebuilding and restoring itself. Sufficient restful sleep helps your body maintain and repair its critical DNA, which will help you replenish skin, muscle, bone and nerve cells as needed. Sleep is very much an anti-inflammation and a pro-longevity lifestyle factor.

One of the most helpful things you can do to relieve inflammation in your body is to increase the consumption of extremely pure water. Fresh, uncontaminated spring water is likely to be the best option. Home-filtering your water with a high quality filter such as the Berky® or the Multi-Pure® is also a viable option. As we stressed in the previous chapter on detoxing, drinking large quantities of water will help dilute the toxins in the natural metabolic inflammatory residue and help flush it from your system. Adding organic lemon juice to your pure water is also helpful because of the detoxifying properties.

Easing into an anti-inflammatory diet is the next obvious step. Remember to consider all processed foods and beverages as inflammatory triggers and try to avoid them. To help in this regard,

I've included the following list of pro-inflammatory foods. If you are aware of or even suspect a food or beverage sensitivity or intolerance, test yourself or have a Clinical Kinesiologist test you for them. Even without that, in general it is better to avoid them.

Foods to Avoid[3]
- Alcoholic beverages
- Artificial sweeteners
- Caffeine
- Chemical additives
- Coffee (including decaf)
- Corn and corn products
- Dairy that is **NOT** pasture raised or organic
- Fast food
- Flour-based foods
- Food preservatives and dyes
- Gluten
- GMO foods
- Margarine
- Packaged and processed foods
- Potatoes
- Red meat (especially if **not** pasture raised or organic)
- Safflower oil
- Shortening
- Spicy foods
- Wheat
- Vegetable oils (except pure, cold pressed olive, flax, macadamia and coconut oils)

Now for the good news! The following is an abbreviated list of foods to include in your diet when combating inflammation. They each have some degree of anti-inflammatory effect. You may also notice that many of these foods are rich in vitamin C, a strong detoxifier and natural inflammation fighter. Remember, choosing organic and non-GMO varieties of these foods further reduces the risk of diet-caused inflammation.

Foods to Include[4]
- Almonds
- Apples
- Avocados
- Blueberries
- Broccoli
- Brussels sprouts
- Butternut squash
- Celery
- Cherries
- Coconut oil
- Cucumbers
- Currants
- Dates
- Flaxseed oil
- Garlic
- Ginger
- Green beans
- Green grapes
- Green tea
- Kale
- Leafy greens
- Herring
- Mackerel
- Mangosteen
- Olive oil
- Oranges
- Persimmons
- Pickles
- Pomegranates
- Prunes
- Quinoa
- Raspberries
- Sardines
- Scallions
- Seaweed
- Tangerines
- Walnuts and walnut oil
- Wild salmon

You may find it helpful to copy these lists and post on your refrigerator, or consult them as you design your shopping list.

Extraordinary Xanthones

Xanthones are naturally-occurring antioxidants with powerful anti-inflammation properties. They have been extensively researched and shown to dramatically reduce inflammation. The tropical fruit, the mangosteen, is the only practical food source. Though many of the powerful anti-inflammatory xanthones are found in the rind of the fruit, which is rarely consumed because of its bitter taste. Historically, people who consumed mangosteen would eat the fruit and dry the rind to make tea. If you are fortunate enough to be living in Southeast Asia you may have an easily available supply, but for the rest of us the mangosteen fruit is impossible to find due to a variety of factors including very specific growing environments and an incredibly short shelf life of approximately three days. So far, all attempts to grow the slow maturing mangosteen trees in North America and Europe have been unsuccessful.

Luckily there is a company that strives to bring the benefit of this unique biochemical substance to people internationally. Xango® juice is available online or through distributors. It is a whole food beverage that combines the whole mangosteen fruit, including the seeds, pericarp and rind, in pureed form with other antioxidant-rich fruit juices and purees. It has no artificial additives or dyes, and no added sugar or water. This product is rich in natural xanthones as well as many other nutrients, and is therefore extremely effective at fighting inflammation. While Xango® juice may seem expensive upon first look; the recommended dosage to achieve maximum health benefits is only one to three ounces per day, which averages to be less than two dollars per serving.

> **A Xango Testimonial**
> Since Consuela had Leaky Gut syndrome (review her story on page 107), her detoxification progress was slow. Her body was rapidly releasing old toxins and making an excess of new toxins each day. Due to the Leaky Gut condition, she reabsorbed many toxins before eliminating them. She decided to have a C-reactive protein blood test done. Her score on this lab test was quite high and she knew she had to jump in to her new natural anti-inflammation program with both feet. Consuela researched the dramatic anti-inflammation effects of the mangosteen fruit and obtained a supply of Xango® juice. After a few months of consuming several ounces of this juice each day, Consuela was convinced that the addition of Xango® juice

had dramatically improved her overall health and had reduced her inflammatory symptoms.

Consuela was able to become more involved in her life and activities and had the energy to maintain a progressively busier schedule. She had a second C-reactive protein blood test after about a year and the results showed that her score had plummeted to the low normal range. Since Consuela's body tended toward inflammatory processes, she continues to drink her xanthone rich, anti-inflammatory Xango® juice and progressively moves forward in her new, healthy life.

Other Anti-Inflammation Nutritional Supplements

A high quality, pure vitamin-C supplement is another natural inflammation-fighter. Quercetin is an effective alternative for inflammation. High doses, 100 to 200 mg daily are often required to squelch acute inflammation. Vitamin B_{12} (methylcobalamin) is effective as well. Omega 3 oils help soothe inflamed tissues and joints. Another inflammation fighter is colostrum.

Digestive Enzymes

If you are not efficiently digesting your food, the oversized particles may contribute to both Leaky Gut syndrome and inflammation. If this is a problem for you, check in with your Clinical Kinesiology practitioner to discover which particular digestive enzyme may be able to help you reduce inflammation. For my patients with chronic inflammation, I recommend a specific digestive enzyme to be taken with or just after meals to foster complete digestion. Additionally, I recommend a different enzyme (a proteolytic enzyme) to be taken separately from meals to assist the body in its cleanup processes. We can liken this enzyme function to adding an algae-eating fish to the metaphorical goldfish tank. (Refer back to Chapter 5, section on Digestive Enzymes.)

Helpful Herbs

Many helpful herbs can decrease or diminish inflammation. These include:

- Aloe
- Burdock root
- Cat's claw
- Celery seed
- Devils claw
- Hawthorne
- Stinging nettles
- Turmeric.

Turmeric, likely the most famous of these, is the herb responsible for the bright yellow color in curries and mustards. Turmeric contains sulfur, that quirky yellow mineral that loves to help you cleanse. You can buy a shaker of organic turmeric in your health food store and use it in many creative ways; for instance, turmeric makes scrambled eggs a much brighter yellow. Make a simple dressing of flaxseed or olive oil, balsamic vinegar, garlic, a few other spices and a liberal amount of turmeric. Add this dressing or plain turmeric to steamed vegetables, soups, salads and stews. The beneficial effects of turmeric are potentiated (bolstered) when it is combined with black pepper and a little bit of fat such as butter, coconut oil or olive oil. Turmeric should also be included in your inflammation-fighting regime. It is available as an herbal supplement in both tincture and capsule form. Taking a supplement of turmeric daily will be beneficial for most inflammation sufferers. Use this remedy twice a day or more if needed.

Sleep: Another Way to Defend Against Inflammation

Another way to defend against problematic inflammation is to allow yourself sufficient rest and sleep. During sleep your body automatically works on detoxifying, rebuilding and restoring itself. Sufficient restful sleep helps your body maintain and repair its critical DNA, which will help you replenish skin, muscle, bone and nerve cells as needed. Sleep is very much an anti-inflammation and a pro-longevity lifestyle factor.

More than just potentiating physical disease, inflammation can also affect your brain function, mood and cognition. We will explore this vital subject in the next chapter.

LEARN MORE
- For a more in-depth description about the inflammatory process and natural ways to approach inflammation you can refer to *Your Body Can Talk,* 2nd Edition, pp. 322-326.
- Refer to *Your Body Can Talk,* 2nd Edition for drug-free approaches to pain on pages 290-293.
- You can read Chapter 8: "Leaky Gut Syndrome" in *Your Body Can Talk, 2nd Edition* to learn more about the insidious development of whole body, toxic inflammation caused by Leaky gut syndrome.
- For a more in-depth description about diabetes and natural ways to approach it, you can refer to *Your Body Can Talk,* 2nd Edition, pp. 310-314.
- You can read more about food-sensitivity testing on pages 105-109 in *Your Body Can Talk, 2nd Edition.*
- You can read more about alcohol and fertility, and Vitamin A deficiency on page 245 of *Your Body Can Talk, 2nd Edition.*
- For more about the incidence of asthma in children whose mothers and grandmothers smoked tobacco, please read pages 243-244 in *Your Body Can Talk, 2nd Edition.*

Books

Babb, Michelle, M.S. R.D. *Anti-Inflammatory Eating Made Easy: 75 Recipes and Nutrition Plan.* Seattle, Wash.: Sasquatch Books, 2014.

Daniluk, Julie. *Meals that Heal Inflammation: Embrace Healthy Living and Eliminate Pain One Meal at a Time.* Carlsbad, Calif.: Hay House, 2011.

Hass, Amanda. *The Anti-Inflammation Cookbook: The Delicious Way to Reduce Inflammation and Stay Healthy.* San Francisco: Chronicle Books, LLC, 2015.

Vasey Christopher, N.D. *Natural Remedies for Inflammation.* Rochester, Vermont: Healing Arts Press, 2013.

Products

Xango® Juice: http://mymangosteen.com/DrSusan/product/juice_xango.asp

Endnotes, Chapter 7

1. Shacter, Emily and Sigmund A. Weitzman. "Chronic Inflammation and Cancer." *Oncology:* January 31, 2002. http://www.cancernetwork.com/review-article/chronic-inflammation-and-cancer
2. Levy, Susan L. *Your Body Can Talk, 2nd Edition*. Chino Valley, Ariz: Kalindi Press, 2014. 146.
3. Ibid, 324.
4. Idem.

CHAPTER 8

Brain Longevity

For many of us, the most frightening concern about moving into our elder years is that we may experience impairments of memory, thinking and decision-making. The good news is that you have already read, and hopefully incorporated into your lifestyle, the essential habits needed to minimize or avoid cognitive decline! Of course, incorporating these habits early in life provides the greatest level of protection. Additionally, you can help to establish more family traditions that encourage each generation to realize and take ownership of the keys to their own health.

Understanding the components and nutritional factors involved in your own body's composition, coupled with common sense detoxification principles and surefire anti-inflammation guidelines, constitutes the best brain-health protection possible.

THE RISK FACTORS OF COGNITIVE DECLINE
Let's begin by looking at a list of the lifetime risk factors for cognitive decline. Most of these are familiar terms, common risk factors that you have likely heard or read about before.
1. Stroke
2. Mild traumatic brain injury (MTBI)
3. Concussion
4. Long-term depression
5. Long-term statin use
6. Alcohol overuse
7. Cardiovascular disease
8. Midlife occurrence of high blood pressure

9. Genetic predisposition
10. Psychotropic prescription drug use
11. Diabetes
12. Loss of sense of smell[1]
13. Eating disorders, especially bulimia

Some of these factors are controllable, and some are not. But, fortunately, many more controllable factors have been identified in recent research. Scientists are finding that nutritional deficiencies contribute to cognitive decline in ways that many of us have been unaware. Below is a list of some of these risk factors that you may not have previously anticipated.

1. Poor nutrition
2. High homocysteine level (confirmed by laboratory test)
3. Toxic metal overload (lead, mercury, aluminum, cobalt, etc.)
4. Mineral excess (or imbalance) especially copper, zinc and iron (classified as transition metals on periodic chart)
5. Micronutrient deficiencies
    A. Vitamins
        1. Vitamin C
        2. Vitamin E complex (tocopherols and tocotrienols)
        3. Vitamin D_3
        4. Vitamin B_{12} (methylcobalamin)
        5. Vitamin B_9 (folic acid)
        6. Vitamin B_1 (thiamine)
        7. Vitamin B_3 (niacin)
        8. Vitamin B_6 (pyridoxine)
    B. Minerals
        1. Selenium
        2. Magnesium
        3. Iron
        4. Manganese
6. Macronutrient deficiency
    A. Essential fatty acids (EFA, especially omega-3)

B. Amino acids
   1. Glutathione
   2. Aminobutyric Acid (GABA)
   3. Glutamate
   4. Aspartate
   5. Glycine

Your Diet Affects Your Brain
These risk factors for cognitive decline, listed above, reflect undeniably that you *are* what you eat, and what you *absorb*. We need a diet of fresh unadulterated, unprocessed, untreated, GMO-free, pesticide free, authentic foods. Fulfilling these conditions, you are supplying your entire body (including your brain) with the necessary fuel and nutrients to sustain and to repair itself. When you realize that environmental toxins, toxic metals, chemical food additives, sugar, food processing technologies and the like, are methods of introducing inflammatory and toxic foreign substances into your body, it will be much easier to select the most brain-protective foods and beverages.

WHAT DOES MY BRAIN LOOK LIKE?

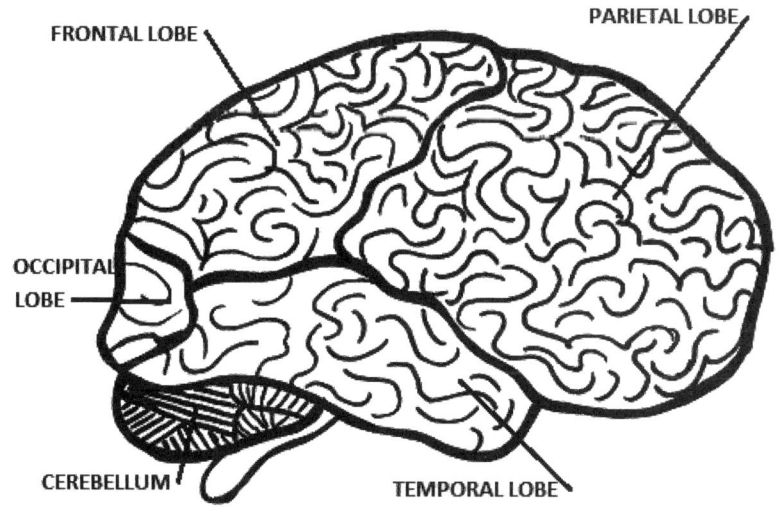

Your brain looks much like the shape and configuration of a walnut, although quite a bit bigger! It has numerous convoluted folds that give it the walnut-like appearance. The cerebrum is the largest portion of your brain; it is your thinking and data storage area. When you are doing any type of thinking, remembering, problem solving and/or purposeful physical activity, you are calling on the cerebrum to guide you.

The outer surface of the cerebrum consists of grey matter commonly referred to as the "cortex." For the most part, sensory input from your five senses (smell, touch, sight, hearing and taste) is processed and interpreted in the cerebral cortex. The cortex is approximately ¼ inch (3.2 mm) thick. Your cerebral cortex is your memory-filing area and is dramatically folded and convoluted to provide a greater surface area.

Your brainstem is composed of three segments that help with your "primitive" or automatic processes. For example, the brainstem regulates breathing, heart rate, kidney function and digestion. It connects the brain to the spinal cord. All sensory and motor pathways going to and from the brain to the body pass through your brainstem. The motor and sensory pathways cross over in your brainstem. This is why the right side of your cerebrum controls the left half of your body and the left half of your cerebrum controls the right half of your body.

If you are like most people, your brain likely weighs approximately 3 pounds (1.5 kilograms). Your brain is highly vascularized, meaning that it is richly supplied with blood by countless arteries and capillaries. In fact, with each heartbeat, approximately twenty percent of blood must go to your brain, since it requires twenty percent of your total oxygen supply. This is one reason why many people with mild memory difficulty or early dementia respond to supplemental or therapeutic oxygen.

HOW DOES MY MEMORY WORK?
Neurons are your body's nerve cells. All of your peripheral nerves (nerves outside the brain that go to the arms legs and torso) are long strands of many neurons linked together. Your peripheral nerves have either motor (movement) or sensory functions, and connect to the spinal cord, sending or receiving their messages to or from your brain.

Within your brain you have at least 100 billion neurons. Each of these nerve cells in your brain connects to at least 10,000 other cells. The amazing fact of all those connections is that you have at least 1000 trillion synapses (nerve connections) in your brain.

Your nervous system creates electricity that moves messages up and down your nerve pathways. Every time a memory is created and transported for storage, the message moves from the long arm of one nerve cell to the next, and then on to the next, by means of body-generated electricity or a combination of electricity and chemical (neurotransmitter) function. As you have new experiences or learn new information, additional linkages (synapses) between your nerve cells are created. If you take good care of your brain, this process can go on throughout your lifetime, and you can store more information and create more folds on the surface of your brain. Ultimately, more and more folds or convolutions are needed to accommodate the information storage as you add data to your memory banks.

After digesting and processing dietary proteins, a variety of amino acids are liberated in your system. Your wise body reassembles specific combinations of amino acids to build each neurotransmitter. Each nerve cell has one long axon (a long thin arm) and multiple dendrites (shorter connecting arms that look like tree branches). Nerve transmission travels along your neuron's arms and branches, incrementally synapsing (connecting) with more and more neurons along the pathway.

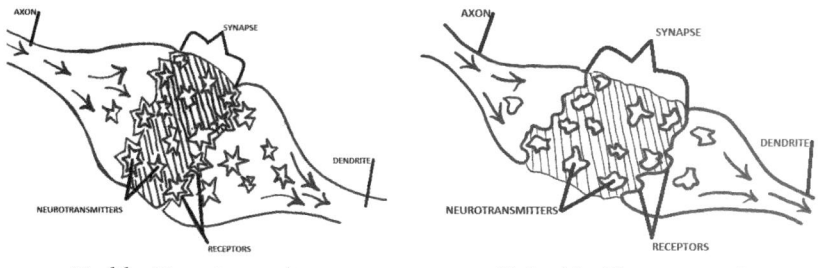

Healthy Neurotransmitter   Unhealthy Neurotransmitter

Besides being protected within its hard bony covering, the cranium, your brain is covered by three layers of protective tissue called the meninges. The meninges extend all the way down your spine covering and protecting the spinal cord as well as the brain. If inflammation or infection enters the meninges and the fluid they hold, the resulting health condition is called meningitis. The fluid contained inside your meninges is called cerebral spinal fluid.

CEREBRAL SPINAL FLUID: YOUR BRAIN'S YOUTH ELIXER
Your cerebral spinal fluid bathes your entire central nervous system, your brain and spinal cord. There are certain nutrients and body constituents in this fluid that need to be present in the correct quantities and ratios. One important function of the cerebral spinal fluid is that it suspends your brain in a protective liquid, simulating a near weightless state. This protects the brain to some degree during a concussion.

In 2012, researchers at Stony Brook University School of Medicine (New York) discovered an additional function of your cerebral spinal fluid. It actually assists your body in flushing away and disposing of toxins created by or otherwise surrounding your brain. This equates to the function of your lymphatic system in all other parts of your body. During this research project, led by Dr. Benveniste, it was determined that the brain did in fact have a very small and delicate set of lymph-like vessels named the "glymphatic system." The glymphatic fluid collects wastes and toxins from the brain and dumps them into your cerebral spinal fluid, which then dissipates through your system.[2] This process only works during sleep and optimally functions primarily during your non-REM 3 sleep stage. When you are resting, most particularly sleeping, all of your brain cells actually shrink dramatically in size. This allows the cleansing fluid to "wash" each cell and sweep out cellular and metabolic debris. The Stony Brook University researchers further discovered that this system works most efficiently while you are lying on your side during sleep. It was specifically found that excess amounts of metabolic protein, believed to cause Alzheimer's disease, is effectively washed away by your well-functioning glymphatic system during a full night's sleep.[3] This further reinforces the better health principle of achieving sufficient sleep and rest. One ironic fact is that Alzheimer's medication is known to be a sleep-disturbing agent.

COGNITIVE IMPAIRMENT
What Is It?

When a person is experiencing any form of dementia or cognitive impairment, there is a lack of efficient electrical and/or chemical transmission of nerve messages in their brain. Terminology to describe cognitive dysfunction is evolving and ever-changing. The term "senility" referred to a deterioration of body and mind associated with advanced aging. This term was too general and now is basically outdated, so it will be avoided in our discussions. "Dementia" is the broad term now used to describe several manifestations of cognitive impairment. The entire field of the neurosciences, which study the dementias, is truly in its infancy. New facts and understandings of the brain and its functions, as well as its disorders, will undoubtedly continue to be discovered.

Currently (2017), we understand that some temporary or totally-reversible forms of dementia exist. These are documented to be caused by specific nutrient deficiencies, by medication side-effects or multiple-drug interactions. As these forms of dementia are easily remedied, we will not focus on them here. Our concern will be with two other groups: non-specified dementias, and dementias stemming from neurodegenerative processes.

In simple terms, each neurodegenerative process is a progressive breakdown or degradation of a person's central nervous system (brain and spinal cord). We can all look forward to the future when more definitive research concerning these conditions has been accomplished. Currently, there is not a simple direct answer as to what actually causes these disorders or what treatments are most appropriate. These specifically named neurodegenerative diseases include Creutzfeldt-Jakob disease, Huntington's disease, Parkinson's disease, and Alzheimer's disease. Here we will briefly consider the non-specified dementia more commonly termed "mild cognitive impairment" (MCI), and actual Alzheimer's disease together.

Cognitive impairment of any type is typically a progressive reduction in brain function. This is first observed by friends, family and coworkers when they compare a person's current mental focus and continuity of memory to those functions in previous years. The family member or helpful close associate will likely notice mild changes long before the affected person realizes that anything is different. Sometimes, the person undergoing mild memory and cognitive change will be defensive and un-accepting of well-intended feedback. These circumstances may delay the person in seeking evaluation or help.

Throughout the time that these symptoms are occurring and progressing, the **beta-amyloid proteins** in the person's brain are building up and adhering to the cerebral cortex faster than they are being detoxified and flushed away. Additionally, another protein malformation is the transformation of **tau proteins** into **neurofibrillary tangles**. Both of these are biochemical and physiological changes characteristic of Alzheimer's disease. The Alzheimer's Association has an informative and easily accessed website (http://www.alz.org/). They have posted warning signs that may indicate Alzheimer's disease.

Beta-amyloid is a naturally-occurring substance, a form of protein that exists in the cortex of most human brains. It seems to be more prevalent and likely to form plaques or clumps that stick to the cortex in those with toxic metal overload, particularly aluminum, mercury and copper. Newer research demonstrates that this beta-amyloid protein protects the brain from heavy metals, pathogenic bacteria, viruses and spirochetes (small organisms akin to bacteria known to be the causative agents for syphilis and Lyme's disease). Some researchers contest the concept that the beta-amyloid actually precipitates the damage to the brain. They believe that this body protein has been called into the brain in greater quantities in order to protect the delicate tissues from an excess of toxic metals and/or pathogenic organisms. That debate will likely continue for years to come.[4]

Regardless of what the debate ultimately proves, incorporating healthy detoxification measures will remain a proactive brain-protecting plan. Seeking a "toxic-metals evaluation" from your natural healthcare practitioner is an excellent first-step strategy. If parasites or a concerning level of toxicity are found by appropriate testing, your natural healthcare practitioner can direct you to suitable treatments for dealing with these conditions, and thereby preserving your memory.

The Risk Busters
All the healthy lifestyle factors that we have considered thus far are general means to protect and enhance our brains as we age. The harmful lifestyle factors that I have encouraged you to avoid also affect every neurodegenerative process or version of dementia. In this next section, we will consider some of the most important ways in which you can decrease your risk of cognitive decline. As you consider each one, I will encourage you to form a strategic plan to minimize as many of these risks as possible.

Cognitive Decline Risk Buster #1:
Stroke and Heart Disease Prevention
Stroke prevention and heart-health measures will automatically improve your overall health and thereby protect your brain. Let's review three preventive actions, starting with avoiding tobacco, trans-fats and chlorinated water. These three are simple steps for many of us. This may be harder for those with certain lifelong habits. But, as I have seen from years as a health practitioner, it is always possible for a person to change when the goal is positive and held clearly in sight.

Including nutrient-rich foods in your diet, rather than devitalized food, is another dynamic measure. An interesting, little-known fact, discovered decades ago, is that eating raw carrots daily is a highly effective way to prevent a stroke.[5] Celery, eggplant, fava beans, Swiss chard and walnuts are a few of the other invaluable blood-pressure balancing (and blood vessel protecting) foods.

And do not forget the herbs and spices! Adding cinnamon, garlic, ginger and turmeric to your foods will not only spice up your meals, but protect your blood vessels, your heart and your brain. These substances are famous for their brain-enhancing qualities. The herbs hawthorn and stinging nettles can be of help. Making your own salad dressing from flaxseed oil and garlic is brain supportive.

Even if you've already had one or more strokes, these measures can improve your life and help to protect you from further incidents.

As you implement the good factors and eliminate the not so good, keep in mind that statin drugs deplete your body's coenzyme Q10. This can weaken several to all of the muscles in your body, particularly your heart, and could result in heart disease that may not have occurred otherwise. Statin drugs are extensively overprescribed today, and are associated with many new cases of diabetes and Alzheimer's disease that were not present in the individual before a long-term course of medication. If you are taking statin drugs please be aware of the risks; study about the consequences and discuss them with your pharmacist and prescribing doctor.

Cognitive Decline Risk Buster #2: Head Injury Prevention

One of the most basic safety concerns for humans at all ages is fall prevention and methods to deter head injuries. Finally, it is a culturally-embraced norm to help fit toddlers with small helmets as they learn to ride their tricycles outdoors. For many people in their elder years, however, helmets were not commonly seen for sporting or hard labor activities during their younger years. Now is the time to consider a helmet or head protection for any activities that include a faster-than-walking pace and a potential for falling.

I urge you to take care to mitigate fall risks in the home, on your sidewalks, porches and in the workplace. If you suffer a fall or a head injury, do not brush it off as minor until you have been evaluated. Seek a medical evaluation to determine the appropriateness of brain imaging that actually could be life saving.

My editor Regina (age 70+) and her husband Jerome (age 80+) keep an Arnica gel and homeopathic Arnica at hand for any bangs and bumps, bruising, falls or trauma. They begin taking Arnica soon after any incident and continue taking it frequently until all symptoms and all pain have resolved. It really works!

Cognitive Decline Risk Buster #3: Depression and Mood Disorders Relief

If you suffer from long-term depression or a mood disorder, this is not a natural accompaniment of aging. While ups and downs (good days and difficult days) are part of life, a grey cloud hovering consistently over your life is not a healthy condition. If this is true for you, it's time to seek professional help. And, at the same time, many natural proactive strategies that *are* under your control will benefit you in your quest. Here are a few simple ideas:

- Avoid alcohol, tobacco, caffeine and sugar because these contribute to emotional volatility.
- Do your best to increase your physical activity.
- Consider one or more activities that connect you with a group of people with similar interests, to increase social interaction. You can busy yourself by becoming involved in more constructive activities. You may want to enroll in self-enrichment classes, courses or groups.
- If you jump into volunteering for a cause or group near and dear your heart, your personal satisfaction level will be elevated.
- Take regular doses of vitamin D_3, a proven mood booster. You can rely on safe sun exposure for a for portion of your daily vitamin D dose, but supplementing with a pure and natural vitamin D_3 supplement in a reasonably high dose (I often recommend 5000 international units daily) will raise your mood and happiness level noticeably.
- Boosting your consumption of vitamins, minerals and amino acids will benefit your brain and therefore your mood. Check in with your natural healthcare provider to help design an individualized program.

If you are actively involved in psychotherapy, counseling or another form of treatment, talk about these suggestions with your healthcare practitioner and ask them for additional natural suggestions.

Cognitive Decline Risk Buster #4: Avoid Substance Abuse

Substance abuse is a significant problem in almost all sectors of modern society. An article about elder substance abuse published in the journal *Addiction,* in 2008, stated that 2.8 million Americans over age 50 were active substance abusers. This study predicted that, by the year 2020, that number would rise to be 5.7 million active substance abusers in the same age bracket.[6]

For elders, one reason for this is an excess of leisure time without a constructive outlet for their energy. Another factor is low self-esteem. Some older aged substance-abusers feel that life has not gone well. They have become emotionally stuck, feeling unable to move forward. As they try to mask their unresolved emotional pain, they may perpetually rely on the short-term elevated endorphin effect from alcohol, opiates or other substances.

> *Endorphins are chemical compounds produced in the pituitary gland; they mimic the action of opiates and produce feelings of pleasure, well-being, and relief from pain…Problem drinkers might experience a subjectively greater "high" compared to social drinkers as the result of increased endorphin activity in critical regions of their brains. This might at least partly account for their propensity to drink greater amounts of alcohol than social drinkers.*[7]

Often, a person in a substance-abuse cycle does not have the foresight or motivation to seek a concrete and long-term solution.

Long-term alcohol overuse does lead to alcoholic dementia. When it is an advanced case it is termed Wernicke-Korsakoff syndrome. At this point dementia and whole-body neuromuscular degeneration are present, along with significant liver damage.

Regardless of the degree or duration of the substance abuse it must stop if brain function is to be preserved. The first step for a person with this issue is to acknowledge that their substance use is out of control. This is not easy, and sometimes requires the intervention of friends and family. The next step is to seek professional help. Many effective programs exist today and are specifically designed to support elders. Betty Ford centers and Alcoholics Anonymous are two well-known rehabilitation centers that have programs specifically geared toward the elder population. Essentially, all of the information and suggestions in minimizing the risks of depression and mood disorders (Risk Buster #3) will apply here.

Cognitive Decline Risk Buster #5: Prevent or Curb Diabetes

Since at least 2008, some neuroscientists and diabetes researchers have been toying with the concept of declaring Alzheimer's disease to be diabetes type III.[8] This is because both disorders have several similar characteristics. Both of these disorders have an excess of the particular protein called beta amyloid-42 and its precursor protein. Both disorders demonstrate other protein molecule dysfunctions, including that of insulin, its related growth factor, and others. Impaired signaling and utilization of insulin by the brain is commonly found in Alzheimer's research studies.

While all of these technical factors are being researched, the undeniable fact remains that the presence of diabetes type 2 is a risk factor for the development of Alzheimer's disease. If you have a family history of diabetes, have been considered pre-diabetic, or diagnosed with diabetes, know that everything you do to be kind to your pancreas and to balance your blood sugar will ultimately benefit your brain health. You will want to avoid processed foods particularly flour-based products and sweetened products to foster your total health picture and preserve your brain's best level of functioning.

You already know that you, like all humans, are genetically geared to search out sweet flavors, but the challenge is to search out and use unprocessed, natural, whole foods in the proper balance with proteins and fats. Apples, oranges, peaches, strawberries, raspberries and other luscious fruits should be eaten slowly and savored. Let these and similarly innocent, unprocessed fruits satisfy your sweet-seeking taste buds.

Once you have wholeheartedly removed processed sweeteners such as sugar, fructose, dextrose, corn sweeteners, high fructose corn sweeteners and the like, your taste buds can once again become realistic. You will need to be a proficient label reader. However, your best food choices will be whole, fresh foods that do not require labels. A wonderful handbook that I highly recommend is *Diabetes without Drugs* by Suzy Cohen, R. Ph. You should find the book to be both enjoyable and informative.

Almonds, avocados, blueberries, unsweetened coconut, coconut oil, eggs, oat bran and oatmeal, unsweetened nut butters, pears, sweet potatoes, turkey, walnuts and wild-caught salmon are healthy foods compatible with your need to balance your blood sugar. Purified water or spring water should be your beverage of choice. Always avoid sweetened beverages whether sugar, fructose or artificial sweeteners are used.

> **Balance Your Blood Sugar with "J-Chokes"**
>
> Look for Jerusalem artichokes; they are nothing like the familiar green globe artichoke. Jerusalem artichokes (a sweet tasting root) are found in your produce section only a few weeks out of the year. These can be sliced and steamed with other vegetables. They taste similar to water chestnuts and directly help balance your blood sugar. I typically slice the fresh harvest of Jerusalem artichokes and dehydrate them for future use. The dried slices are a wonderful substitute for chips and you can dip them into hummus or guacamole with no blood sugar spike. Anytime you want to make a soup or stew you can add half a cup of the dried chips. They will seem similar to potatoes by the time they're cooked. You can use them as a potato substitute in many recipes.
>
> To have a sustainable supply of Jerusalem artichokes, it is best to grow them yourself. They will grow in almost any temperate climate and are both prolific and invasive. I suggest segregating them to a specific garden bed, a raised bed or a large container. Jerusalem artichokes are available in your grocery store or health food store. You can buy a pound or two, use half for consumption and plant the rest. The roots will look similar to a ginger root and often have little buds or knobs that you can separate and plant individually. During the growing season, they will put out tall spires of green foliage that typically flower at the very end of the growing season with a small sunflower-type bloom. When the foliage has died back, it's time to dig out the roots with a garden fork. Once you have cleaned and dried your Jerusalem artichokes you can either store them in the refrigerator for months or dehydrate them.

Cognitive Decline Risk Buster #6: Avoid Sleep Deficiency

There is nothing more restorative to your brain than a good night's sleep. One of your best brain-health protectors is to consistently treat yourself to sufficient quality sleep. Doing your best to adhere to a reasonable and consistent schedule for going to sleep and getting up is the foundation for good sleep. There are also many other practices, which I will enumerate below, that will aid you in getting the best rest and sleep possible.

- Avoid caffeine after 2:00 P.M.
- Avoid snacking after dinner to allow your digestive system to naturally perform and then wind down.
- Give your entire body and mind an hour or more to wind down before bedtime. You may find that you are able to get to sleep more quickly.
- Create a new relaxing and sleep-inducing routine: drink chamomile, oat straw tea, or another relaxing tea while reading a book, have meaningful interaction with your spouse and/or family, or while spending a little time with your favorite craft or hobby rather than watching the nightly news or an intense action movie.
- Organic dairy products sourced from grass-fed cows and turkey meat contain tryptophan, a sleep inducing amino acid.
- Be sure to do tomorrow's planning and finish today's problem-solving in a different part of the house before going to your bedroom for the night.
- Avoid interacting with your electronic devices for at least an hour or two before bedtime.
- Be sure that your bedroom is free from sources of electromagnetic pollution. Do not have computers, televisions or charging stations in your bedroom.

Some people have disturbed sleep patterns because they need to get up during the night to use the bathroom. If the urinary frequency relates to a health issue such as enlarged prostate, learning about natural remedies and noninvasive help would be the first logical step. Consulting with your doctor or natural healthcare practitioner will be the next step. If your nighttime urination is not due to a health issue, you may be able to train yourself to go back to sleep with ease by using meditation or another method. If this is not feasible and you find it too difficult to go back to sleep after waking up to use the bathroom, you may choose to have a bedside receptacle or even a bedside commode in your bedroom in order to avoid a trip to the bathroom that leads you down a hall or requires navigating stairs. Another option is to limit your liquid or water intake in the evenings so that you can postpone nighttime bathroom trips until morning.

Cognitive Decline Risk Buster #7: Nutrition for Your Brain
Remember that your brain is composed of delicate tissues that perform amazing tasks around the clock. When you are engrossed in extremely focused study, critical thinking, concentration or problem solving, you can use much more than the typical amount of your body's available energy for your cerebral functions. Your brain thrives on the glucose that your body has broken down from your macronutrient intake. It is vital that your entire body, and most especially your brain, has a consistent and full supply of all essential nutrients, vitamins, minerals, unaltered carbohydrates, proteins and essential fatty acids.[9] When it comes to your brain health, processed foods, food additives and sugary sweet junk can be detrimental and even poisonous. It goes without saying, therefore, that your best line of defense is a good offense.

Throughout your life, all of your neurons can grow longer arms and branches and make new connections (synapses) with other neurons. All of this requires energy and nutrients, even while you are sleeping. One **vitamin necessary for the health** of your brain and entire nervous system is vitamin B_{12}.[10] Chronic vitamin B_{12} deficiency can result in a temporary state of dementia along with nerve dysfunction and even disabling muscle weakness.

Numerous **amino acids are necessary** to create the neurotransmitters that help transmit messages and electrical impulses up and down your numerous nerve pathways. (You can review Chapter 5, page 92, for more information on this.) Your memory and nervous system are further optimized by other beneficial nutrients that may not be considered classically essential. Examples of these include **nonessential amino acids** such as **acetyl L carnitine**[11] and **L- carnosine** that are both considered to be rejuvenators for your body and particularly for your brain.

Glycerophosphorylcholine has shown promising benefit to individuals who have had transient ischemic attacks, strokes, drug-induced amnesia and neurotransmitter deficiency. This brain builder is available in capsules or powder in combination with other brain building nutrients and is often recommended in 400 mg per day dosage.

Phosphatidyl serine is classified as a phospholipid. You may recall that phospholipids are prevalent in all of your cell membranes, including your brain tissues. Phosphatidyl serine has been shown to improve memory, mood, concentration, stress coping, and may even help restore language skills that have been diminished by dementia. Phosphatidyl serine is also available in capsules and powder form and is often recommended in dosages between 120 and 250 mg per day. When it comes to your brain, it would be best to supply yourself with more than the baseline of necessary nutrients than to be even a little bit deficient in any one of them.

The next chapter, *Youthing for Health and Longevity* is truly a culmination of everything discussed thus far in this book. It is my sincere hope that you will find encouragement and inspiration to use your own creative process in approaching youthing.

LEARN MORE
- For a deeper understanding about your natural sleep stages and how to achieve better quality sleep, you may refer to pages 336-342 in *Your Body Can Talk, 2nd Edition.*
- For more understanding of prostate difficulties and do-it-yourself tips to help your prostate gland, read pages 227-232 in *Your Body Can Talk, 2nd Edition.*
- To learn more about stroke prevention, read pages 327-331 in *Your Body Can Talk, 2nd Edition.*
- Refer to pages 300 and 301 *in Your Body Can Talk, 2nd Edition* for more proactive ways to protect your blood vessels, your heart, prevent strokes and maintain good cognitive function.

- To learn more about natural ways to balance your blood pressure, read pages 315-321 in *Your Body Can Talk, 2nd Edition*
- For more in-depth coverage and to find natural ways to help relieve depression you can review pages 303-309 in *Your Body Can Talk, 2nd Edition.*
- For a more in-depth description about diabetes and natural ways to approach it, you can refer to *Your Body Can Talk, 2nd Edition's* pages 310-314.
- You may want to refer to pages 174-178 in *Your Body Can Talk, 2nd Edition* for more tips on reducing electromagnetic pollution in your home.

Books

Babb, Michelle, MS, RD, CD. *Anti-Inflammatory Eating for a Happy, Healthy Brain: 75 Recipes for Improving Depression, Anxiety, and Memory Loss.* Seattle, Wash.: Sasquatch Books, 2016.

Carney, Colleen, Ph.D. and Rachel Manber, Ph.D. *Quiet Your Mind and Get to Sleep: Solutions to Insomnia for Those with Depression, Anxiety or Chronic Pain.* Oakland, Calif.: New Harbinger Publications, Inc., 2009.

Cohen, Gene D., M.D., Ph.D. *The Mature Mind: The Positive Power of the Aging Brain.* Cambridge, Mass.: Basic Books, 2006.

Cohen, Suzy R. Ph. *Diabetes without Drugs: The 5-Step Program to Control Blood Sugar Naturally and Prevent Diabetes Complications.* Emmaus, Penn.: Rodale Inc., 2010.

Denton, Gail L., Ph.D., *Brainlash: Maximize Your Recovery from Mild Brain Injury,* Third Edition. New York: Demos Medical Publishing, 2008.

Mason, Douglas J., PSY. D. *The Mild Traumatic Brain Injury Workbook: Your Program for Regaining Cognitive Function and Overcoming Emotional Pain.* Oakland, Calif.: New Harbinger Publications, Inc., 2004.

Smith, Fraser, B.A., M.A.T.D., N.D. *The Complete Brain Exercise Book: Train Your Brain—Improve Memory, Language, Motor Skills and More.* Toronto: Robert Rose, 2015.

Websites
The Alzheimer's Association: http://www.alz.org

Endnotes, Chapter 8
1. Wesson, Daniel W., Efrat Levy, Ralph A. Nixon and Donald A. Wilson. "Olfactory Dysfunction Correlates with Amyloid- Burden in an Alzheimer's Disease Mouse Model." *The Journal of Neuroscience.* 30:2 (January 13, 2010). 505-214
2. "Brain May Flush Out Toxins During Sleep." *National Institutes of Health.* Accessed August 18, 2015. http://www.nih.gov/news/health/oct2013/ninds-17.htm
3. "Lack of Sleep Promotes Alzheimer's by Preventing Critical Detoxification." *Mercola.* Accessed August 18, 2015. http://articles.mercola.com/sites/articles/archive/2015/04/02/poor-sleep-promotes-alzheimers.aspx
4. "Microbes Implicated in Alzheimer's." *Royal Society of Chemistry.* March 23, 2010. http://www.rsc.org/chemistryworld/News/2010/March/23031003.asp
5. Carper, Jean. *Food—Your Miracle Medicine: How Food Can Prevent and Cure Over 100 Symptoms and Problems.* New York: Harper Collins Publishers, 1993, 8.
6. Han, Beth, Joseph C. Gfroerer, James D. Colliver and Michael A. Penne. "Substance Use Disorder Among Older Adults in the United States in 2020." *Addiction.* 104:1 (January 2009), 88-96.
7. George, Simon, PhD. "Alcohol and Endorphins: 'Feel Good' Chemical Key to Problem Drinking?" *Counseling Resource: Psychology, Philosophy and Real Life.* Accessed August 31, 2015. http://counsellingresource.com/features/2012/01/18/endorphins-and-alcohol/
8. De la Monte, Suzanne M., M.D., M.P.H. and Jack R. Wands, M.D. "Alzheimer's Disease is Type 3 Diabetes—Evidence Reviewed." *Journal of Diabetes Science and Technology.* 2:6 (November 2008), 1101-1113.
9. Gu, Yian, Ph.D., Jeri W. Nieves, Ph.D., Yaakov Stern, Ph.D., Jose A. Luchsinger, M.D., M.P.H., and Nikolas Scarmeas, M.D., M.S. "Food Combination and Alzheimer Disease Risk: A Protective Diet." *The Journal of American Medical Association.* 67:6 (June 2010), 699-706.
10. Clarke, Robert, M.D., David Smith, DPhil, Kim A. Jobst, D.M., Helga Refsum, M.D., Lesley Sutton, BSc and Per M. Ueland, M.D. "Folate, Vitamin B12, and Serum Total Homocysteine Levels in Confirmed Alzheimer Disease." *The Journal of American Medical Association.* 55:11 (November 1998), 1449-1455.
11. Pettegrew, Jay, W., William E. Klunk, Kanagasabai Panchalingam, Julian N. Kanfer and Richard J. McClure. "Clinical and Neurochemical Effects of Acetyl-L-Carnitine in Alzheimer's Disease." *Neurobiology of Aging.* 16:1 (January-February, 1995), 1-4.

CHAPTER 9

Youthing: Create Your Health and Longevity

Youthing: *v. the conscious process of figuratively regressing in age for healthful purposes such as memory enhancement, physical vitality and emotional health; implies the opposite of aging.*

Youthing is characterized by a positive approach to life, philosophically, spiritually, mentally and emotionally. Maintaining flexibility of our body, mind, emotions and habits allows us to glide through our elder years. Clinical Kinesiology and its use of muscle response testing are self-empowering tools to these ends. When we test ourselves we tap into our inner wisdom and become more mindful of our best lifestyle options and choices.

THE POSITIVE APPROACH
Embracing more positive thoughts and using more positive language holds greater benefit than using language and thought patterns that have been corrupted or have negative connotations. Obviously, with the birth of each new day, we each become older, as quantified by the calendar. However, each day that we awaken with a positive outlook, self-acceptance, gratitude for our lives and our gifts, we are "reborn" with fresh human potential. A counterproductive (and inadvisable) way to greet your morning would be to say to yourself "another day older." A more positive and inspiring way to greet your smiling countenance in the mirror would be: "I am ready for the rich adventures that today will bring!" You could follow that with, "I am grateful for my blessings and

my ability to be productive." In essence, every day, you choose whether to consider that your day brings forth a bright horizon of great potential or to lament yesterday's shortcomings.

> *Emerging literature has begun to identify the health benefits of positive emotions. In older populations, studies show that high positive emotion can reduce the risk of incident disability and mobility limitations, stroke, cardiovascular and all-cause mortality, and can aid in recovery from Coronary Artery Bypass Graft surgery. Knowing an older person's emotional well-being prior to a heart attack, stroke or hip fracture is also a good predictor of functional recovery one year post event.[1]*

You can probably relate to the fact that on days when you start out in a good mood and with a positive attitude, generally things go well. Working to constructively create a positive frame of mind and adapt to and overcome minor disappointments enhances your quality of life, promotes your body's structural integrity and promotes longevity.

Maintaining a positive attitude and looking for ways to build and maintain happiness and fulfillment in your life are prerequisites for your personal youthing process.

Mindfulness as a Daily Practice

Becoming more mindful of your life—your actions, your thoughts, your emotions, and how you relate to others brings many benefits. Practicing mindfulness helps us to live in the present moment and to be more aware and engaged in each moment. This, in a sense, allows us to savor life, our thoughts, our perceptions and our experiences. Being focused diverts us from distraction and lets us move beyond "mind chatter," if we are patient.

Beginning your mindfulness practice is as simple as scheduling a ten- or fifteen-minute appointment for yourself with yourself.
- Sit comfortably.
- Allow relaxation to envelop you as you practice slow, relaxed breathing—deeper than normal, but not forced.

- Encourage your mind to slow by focusing on your breath. Remind yourself to stay with the present moment.

Initially, your mind may wander to the past, to tomorrow or to your To-Do list. Gently work to refocus on **now** and your steady, relaxing breath. This process gives you a pause from the rush of everyday life and its challenges.

Benefits of a Mindfulness or Meditation Practice
- Improved immunity
- Improved flexibility
- Improved brain function, including memory and learning
- Better moods and more balanced emotions
- Decreased incidence of depression
- Decreased incidence of agitation
- Increased compassion for others
- Enhanced relationship satisfaction
- Increased acceptance of self, others and circumstances

I prefer to practice mindfulness first and then move to meditation (peaceful concentration on a specific topic or concern). You can learn the Youthing Meditation that I have designed for us all on page 188-190. As you practice mindfulness and explore meditation, you will find yourself adapting to change with greater ease. Including a mindfulness practice in your daily life will help you find your inner wisdom.

Flexibility Extends Youth

Youthing is characterized by the ability to maintain flexibility in every aspect of your life. That is, when plan A does not work, the flexible person smoothly shifts into plan B. Such shifting reflects the ability to handle stress in creative ways.

Stretching, practicing yoga or Tai Chi, walking and staying physically active helps us improve our physical flexibility. Stretching our minds by reading, studying, watching documentaries, taking classes, and learning new languages and new skills are proactive steps for keeping our minds flexible. Even more challenging would be a non-adversarial discussion of controversial topics with your friends, both from your preferred viewpoint, and from the opposite vantage point. Meditation, positive imagery, conscious use of affirmations, and setting and achieving life goals are youthing tools that we can all adapt to enhance our flexibility. Being emotionally flexible is a great stress reducer! According to Ronald Klatz, M.D. and Robert Goldman M.D., world renowned anti-aging specialists:

> *Studies have shown that people with relaxed personalities have a more stable mood and are better able to handle stressful situations without anxiety. They also may be better positioned to prevent age-related cognitive decline… In addition, maintaining a positive outlook and managing stress levels were positive contributors to health with age.*[2]

Full Engagement, Life's Purpose
Committing yourself to being fully engaged in your life will reconnect you to your dynamic *ikigai*. Remember from Chapter 1 that *ikigai* is the Okinawan term for "the reason for which you get up in the morning." Identifying your personalized version of your own reason for being is another important component of your youthing process. This is akin to using your internal compass to stay on your life's path. You are truly free to redesign or redirect your path and your purpose as often as you choose.

Being consciously aware of the depth of *who you truly are* and how you best relate to the fabric of your life, your relationships, your community and your own very personal spiritual or religious path is another step in your youthing process.

THE "MICROCOSM" IN ME
Another concept to consider in this exploration of youthing is "How do I fit into my personal universe?" I consider my personal universe to include several layers, or orbits. (See illustration on page 186.) The most

obvious component of a personal universe is the self—myself or you, yourself. This includes not only the physical body, but the emotional "self" and the spiritual "self." The body-self is composed of smaller units: cells and their organelles and DNA, the vital organs, tissues and bones that form the physical body. The physical body is enlivened by *chi*, the spark of life, the life-force, soul or spirit. Inseparable from our body and our actions is our emotional self. These factors (physical, spiritual, emotional) are unique to each person, and provide our distinctive personality and being.

We will begin our consideration of our own microcosm (miniature world) with a look at the component parts of our physical bodies: our cells, their DNA and their organelles, as well as our life-giving organs.

Restore Your Telomeres: Youth Promoting Components of Your DNA

Organelles are microscopic "organs" inside your cells. Each type of organelle has very specific functions to carry out. Some of those functions are for energy production, maintenance and cellular repair. Other functions include recognizing substances that are compatible with your body, and also identifying and trying to eliminate those that are not. The nucleus ("brain") and the mitochondria ("liver") within your cells contain your DNA, which is necessary for all cellular rebuilding, growth and repair. The protective end-caps on your DNA strands are called **telomeres**. As time progresses, the telomeres more or less erode and ravel, becoming shorter. The length of your telomeres reveals your physiological age and longevity potential. This is distinct from your chronological age that is based on your birth date.

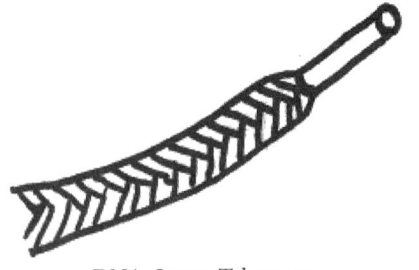
DNA–Intact Telomeres

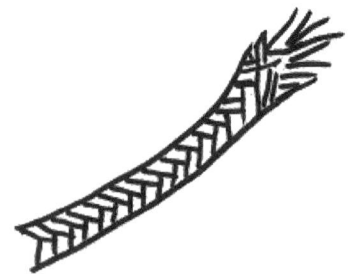
DNA–Frayed Telomeres

In many ways your DNA and telomeres are responsible for both the beginning and the ending of your physical life. If you encourage age-accelerating factors in your lifestyle then your telomeres will shorten prematurely, advance your physiological age and theoretically shorten your lifespan.

Thankfully, you have the option to exclude or diminish age-accelerating factors from your lifestyle. You are free to indulge in health-building and even youthing factors to embellish your health, **to protect and even restore your telomeres.** As you thoughtfully live a youthing lifestyle, you can decrease your physiological age and lengthen your lifespan, while adding quality of life to your years. Of course, many diverse and complicating factors can enter into this equation, but the most logical approach for any of us is to avoid toxic age-accelerating lifestyle factors and to treat our bodies, right down to our telomeres, with the utmost of care, nurturance and respect.

Telomere Supportive Foods
- Asparagus
- Bee pollen
- Blueberries
- Broccoli
- Cantaloupe
- Dark leafy greens
- Grape seeds and grape seed oil
- Green tea
- Nuts and seeds (sources of sulfur)
- Strawberries
- Sweet potatoes
- Tomatoes
- Turmeric

In the years and decades to come, humans will be exposed to more and more helpful information about keeping their telomeres intact and healthy. For now, you can feel confident that all nine chapters of this book are telomere-friendly; they can serve as your guidebook to proper care of your countless telomeres. Following the programs laid out here will promote health and longevity.

A simple, lifestyle-enhancing practice to promote accelerated telomere repair and lengthening is to drink three cups of green tea per day. A research study in 2009 found that this practice promoted longer telomeres in subjects when compared with those of a control group who drank a smaller amount of green tea daily.[3]

Decaffeinated green tea is available for those who want to avoid caffeine. Green tea extract is available in liquid and capsule form.

> **Green Tea and Detox**
> Green tea helps the body to detoxify. Those with high levels of toxicity or those who have not cleansed their system recently may experience an uncomfortable reaction to detoxification. If you experience discomfort, you may need to modify the amount of green tea you consume.

The Chinese herb astragalus has been in use for centuries to assist with immune building and support for cancer patients. Astragalus is known to help diabetics to balance their blood sugar and to help with chronic fatigue. Recent studies have shown astragalus to assist the body in producing telomerase, a critical biological enzyme required to maintain and repair your telomeres.[4]

> **Telomere Supportive Nutrients**[5]
> - Acetyl-L carnitine*
> - All components of the B vitamin complex, especially methylcobalamin (B_{12}) and folate
> - Glutathione
> - L-carnitine*
> - Magnesium
> - Serine*
> - Sulfur
> - Tryptophan*
> - Vitamin C
> - Vitamin E
> - Zinc
>
> *Refer to page 92 in Chapter 5 for more information

Numerous studies document the DNA-strengthening and bolstering effects of these nutrient factors. Some of these even help reverse degradation or shortening of the telomeres. This slows the aging process and promotes youthing. Below are more telomere-supporting actions you can choose to adopt.

> **Lifestyle Factors that Support Telomeres**
> - Reduction of stress
> - Meditation/mindfulness practices
> - Reduction of inflammation
> - Avoidance of smoking and tobacco products
> - Avoidance of alcoholic beverages
> - Regular and sufficient sleep
> - Adoption of health supportive diet as described in Chapter 5
> - Incorporation of detoxification principles in Chapter 6
> - Continuing to be physically, mentally and socially active.
> - Practicing forgiveness and gratitude while loving yourself and others.

I Am Hungry. I Made 300 Billion Cells Today.

The typical adult human body is composed of 100 trillion cells. It busily builds approximately 300 billion new cells daily, since during each minute of life, 300 million old cells die and are sloughed off. This is how your body constantly replenishes cells, tissues and organs, and why a wholesome, nutritious diet is so critically important in maintaining your health. Fresh, raw materials are constantly being used to refurbish your body and its components.

Appreciate Your Miraculous Body

After considering your organelles and cells, let us next consider a sampling of miraculous facts about the important organs that perform all the necessary tasks for your body, as well as the miracles of your blood system, skin and brain.

Your heart, lungs, liver, kidneys, pancreas, thyroid adrenals and digestive tract are constantly replacing and rebuilding themselves. The lining of your gastro-intestinal tract is replaced with new cells at least once per week. Other organs have an infusion of new cells consistently, but at different rates. Your liver replaces all of its cells in cycles of one to two years.

On average, each person has 60,000 miles (96,560.64 kilometers) of blood vessels. This includes arteries, veins, arterioles, veinules, and capillaries. This distance is more than twice the circumference of the earth. This extensive infrastructure brings fresh blood with oxygen and nutrients to each cell in your body approximately once each minute.

Your skin's total surface area is approximately 25 square feet (7.62^2 meters) and contains about 45 miles (72.42 kilometers) of sensory nerves. Twenty feet (6 meters) of blood vessels are contained in each square inch (25^2 millimeters) of your skin. Your skin separates internal body fluids, cells and organs from your external environment and helps create your uniquely personal microbiome (environment of your beneficial bacteria). Skin to skin contact between parents and their newborns helps transfer these healthy (probiotic) bacteria to the infant. This builds the baby's immunity.

The human brain is quite miraculous: containing 100 billion nerve cells with up to 1,000 trillion synapses (transmissive nerve connections). This allows for memory, data storage, critical thinking, and monitoring of thousands of physiological functions, all of which make the human experience possible. Your brain collects and responds to countless messages coming and going to and from all parts of your body tirelessly and with exquisite precision, day in and day out.

Take a moment to appreciate your entire body. In my opinion, the human body is the most miraculous creation in nature. We can think of the body, the human mind, human emotions, goals and endeavors as one harmonious unit, your **self**. I encourage you to research further and learn more of your body's wonders.

I AM PART OF A "MACROCOSM" (A GREATER WHOLE)

Next we can consider how we each relate to others and to the external world around us. We can consider these "outer orbits" of our personal universe to be our macrocosm, the greater reality that we are part of. Every aspect of our self participates in forming our relationships to others, to our community or communities, and to our religious or spiritual beliefs and community.

Building Relationships

The next phase when thinking about how you fit into your universe is to look at the realm of your individual and personal relationships with other people and your pets. Your relationships are critically important to all facets of your well-being. Your relationships require care, "feeding" and your attention in order to thrive.

Previously, we considered the analogy of goldfish in an aquarium to demonstrate the vital need for care of the environment in determining health. Here, we might extend that analogy to see the goldfish in the aquarium as symbolizing relationships. If you recognize that one or more of your important relationships have degenerated because they have been poorly tended, exposed to psychic or emotional toxicity, inadequately "fed," or have somehow been wounded, it is best to properly attend to those issues. Healing and enriching your important relationships will ultimately resolve a lot of discomfort and pain. This may be a challenging and difficult task, but should ultimately be rewarding. Excesses of forgiveness and gratitude are much healthier than deficiencies of compassion and happiness. This is another youthing endeavor.

As you achieve greater balance and health within your body, mind and emotions and have brought comfort to your relationships, you will more easily fit into your larger community or communities. Your interests, hobbies, activities, goals, work and relationships may move you to participate in various specific communities. The act of participating and sharing an aspect of life with a group, or with several groups, will add depth and vibrancy to your life. The positive and meaningful exchanges within a community can actually add years to your life and to the lives of others.

Consider Your Spiritual Life in the Second Half

Another realm to embrace in your own personal way is to be involved in a spiritual or religious community. Each person will choose their path and their level of engagement, and the potential for personal enrichment and sharing is limitless. For centuries, the power of prayer has been demonstrated throughout every culture. Modern research studies have conclusively shown remarkable benefits not only to those being prayed for but also to those who pray for others.[6]

As we mature into wise elders, we may be inspired to reflect on the same spiritual questions that our ancestors pondered: Why are we here? What is the meaning of life? What is the spiritual nature of the universe, of our planet and its inhabitants? Is there life after physical death?

What are your burning questions? Write them down and search for the answers.

Mindfulness, thoughtful awareness, contemplation and meditation have also been beneficial to countless people over many centuries. Engaging in your spiritual or religious practice of choice is a highly-rewarding youthing experience.

USING CLINICAL KINESIOLOGY

Below is a diagram that encompasses these concepts of the personal universe that we have been considering. Studying this diagram and asking yourself (using Clinical Kinesiology) if you feel balanced in each of these areas will help you determine what's working for you and what needs attention. Seeing the big picture may also help you fit a little more comfortably into your personal universe.

My Personal Universe

Organelles — Cells — Organs — Body (Self) — Relationships — Community — Spiritual or Religious Community

To use this illustration, as a guide for self-testing with Clinical Kinesiology, begin by sitting comfortably in a chair, and placing this book in front of you so you can easily see the chart. Do a preliminary indicator muscle test, or have your testing partner do this, to ensure you are ready for other muscle tests. You may want to review the Clinical Kinesiology muscle-testing instructions on pages xvii-xviii in the Introduction. While performing the muscle tests, you or your testing partner can sequentially ask your body these specific questions:

- Are my organelles nourished and balanced?
- Are my cells nourished and balanced?
- Are my organs nourished and balanced?
- Is my body nourished and balanced?
- You can follow these questions with: Is my community participation balanced and nourishing? Again, you may ask individual questions for specific communities that you participate in.
- The last question pertaining to how you relate to your "personal universe" chart should be something like: Is my spiritual community participation balanced and nourishing?

Some may choose to simply consider or contemplate the chart alone or to design other questions.

You should always look for natural and proactive remedies or "fixes" for any out-of-balance orbits in your personal universe. You may decide to periodically revisit these questions and reevaluate your perspective on your personal universe. By addressing neglected or out of balance "orbits" you are paving the way for your youthing lifestyle.

TALK TO YOUR BODY

One of the most important processes you can undertake is to creatively use your own consciousness to talk to your body. Use visual imagery, affirmations and focused meditation. Each one is a powerful tool. Your body wants to hear your positive input. A study conducted by Ellen Langer suggested that "many of the things we consider as inevitable consequences of aging (e.g., diminished energy, physical strength and endurance, memory and other cognitive abilities, etc.) might be significantly influenced by our perceptions and mind-set."[7]

I devised the following Youthing Meditation prior to writing this book. I have faithfully practiced this meditation each morning and truly feel that I have benefited. For myself, I have incorporated giving attention to all joints in my body beginning with the joints between the segments of my toes up through the ankles, knees, hips, sacroiliac, lumbar spine, thoracic spine, cervical spine, shoulders, elbows, wrists and finger joints during this meditation. I have typically told my body to remember and relive being eighteen-to-twenty years old as I focus on each of these joint areas. Generally, I move those joints slightly (in sequence from toes up to fingers) during the meditation to be sure that each area is addressed. I have experienced increased comfort and mobility for most of my joints over the period of actively pursuing this meditation. In addition, I spend time focusing on my body's organs, cells and telomeres. I intend to continue this meditation and I hope you will join me in the Youthing Meditation on a frequent, if not daily, basis. Then you will truly be an expert in the youthing process.

Youthing: A Meditation
This Youthing Meditation can help your cells remember how to grow and replenish themselves in the healthiest and best way possible.
1. Choose a time in your life when you felt the healthiest, strongest and the most balanced and vibrant. Visualize yourself living and feeling very well and healthy. Hold this image in your mind and allow the feeling of wellness to encompass your body. You may chose to incorporate Clinical Kinesiology muscle testing to select an age to visualize, such as 20, 30, 42, etc.
   - For example, if you choose to place yourself in a time *prior* to a specific loss—such as death of a loved one—you will relive that era and regenerate your body, mind and being to a more comfortable time when you were not yet affected by the loss.
   - Another example would be choosing a comfortable time prior to an injury such as a fall, car wreck, fracture, loss of a limb, loss of vision, or loss of any other bodily or mental function.

Youthing: Create Your Health and Longevity 189

- Select a time in your life that you want to re-experience, if that suits you best.
2. Begin by tapping with your fingertips on both the right and left sides of your head at your temples. Do this tapping five or six times while thinking or verbally repeating your selected "target age."
    - Start by tapping your right temple directly in front of your ear canal and continue tapping in an upward motion around the top of your ear all the way around to behind the center of the ear opposite of where you started. Repeat this process on the left temple and going around the left ear. This encourages your nervous system to "reset" to the selected time.
3. Gently tap middle of your forehead three to six times.
4. Lie on your left side in the fetal position. Interlace your fingers and comfortably hold your locked hands slightly above your head. Keep this position for a minimum of three to five minutes, or as long as comfortable.
    - During this time you will be resetting, restoring, remembering, daydreaming, meditating, and or praying. Your goal is to reestablish your health, physiology, feelings, abilities, and sense of well-being to the level that you experienced during the chosen time period of your life.
    - You may choose to focus on a specific body part or multiple areas of the body. Your goal is to "youth" these areas, essentially by turning back the clock.
5. Affirm that you already have the wisdom, experience, balance and foresight of a revered elder.
6. Gently turn over and lie on your right side in the fetal position, repeating or progressing the process described in step 4.
    - Remember to be fluid and self-expressive in your meditation experience.
    - You may focus on the joints while lying on your left, and your organs while lying on your right side.
    - Choose the most comfortable position(s) to lie in for your relaxing meditation.
7. Repeat this Youthing Meditation daily.

- I suggest starting your day with this practice while still in bed. If you should fall asleep, no harm will be done. Your unconscious mind will carry on the healing process during sleep and when you awaken. You will be reinforcing to the conscious mind with the unconscious mind, and your body can again function as it did twenty, thirty, forty, fifty or sixty years ago.

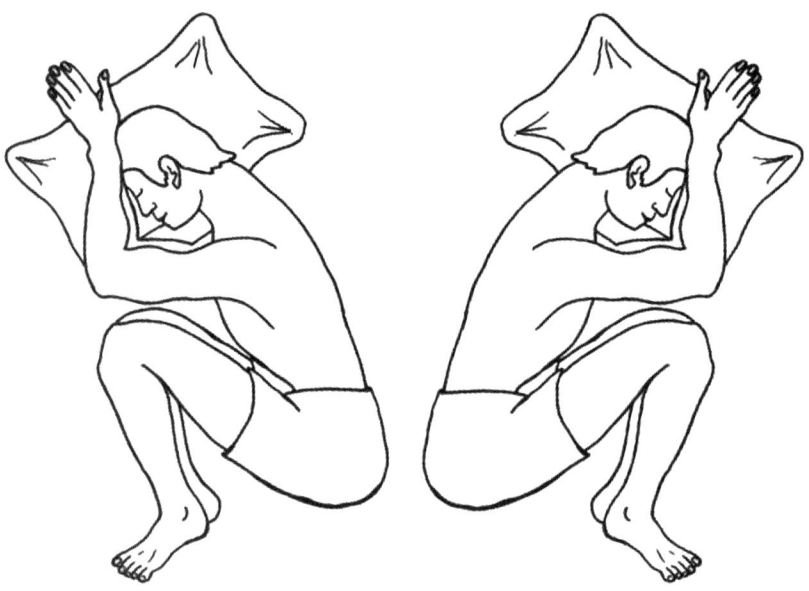

There's still a lot of research to do on the mind-body connection, but if there's one thing all the recent research on aging and the influence of psychological factors tells us, it's that our surroundings, our relationships, our activities, and how we think and feel about our lives really matters. If we're active and engaged, if we place ourselves in "youthful" and energetic surroundings, and immerse ourselves in those surroundings, we tend to feel better, look and feel younger, and age more gracefully.[8]

You have been exposed to an array of youthing tools. Begin using some of these today. You may want to take a little time to study and explore others or consider how to individualize them for yourself. Building your new youthing lifestyle will be rewarding. You can start this process at any age and I suggest you **begin youthing today!**

LEARN MORE
- Review Chapter 3, "Energy and Emotions," pages 54-72, of *Your Body Can Talk, 2nd Edition* by Susan L. Levy, D.C.
- Review The Afterword, "Organ Meditation" on pages 346-348, of *Your Body Can Talk, 2nd Edition* by Susan L. Levy, D.C.

Books

Canfield, Jack and Mark Victor Hansen. *Chicken Soup for the Golden Soul: Heartwarming Stories About People 60 and Over.* Deerfield Beach, Fla.: Health Communications, Inc., 2000.

Chopra, Deepak. *Ageless Body, Timeless Mind: The Quantum Alternative to Growing Old.* New York: Three Rivers Press, 1994.

Davich, Victor. *8 Minute Meditation Expanded: Quiet Your Mind. Change Your Life.* New York: Penguin Group (USA) LLC, 2004.

Goldman, Robert, M.D., D.O. and Ph.D. and Lisa Berger. *Brain Fitness: How to Achieve Super Mind-Power and Keep it as Long as You Live.* New York: Doubleday, 1998.

Kabat-Zinn, Jon. *Coming to Our Senses: Healing Ourselves and the World Through Mindfulness.* New York: Hyperion Books, 2006.

Klatz, Ronald, M.D., D.O. and Robert Goldman, M.D., D.O. and Ph.D. *121 Ways to Live 121 Years and More!: Prescriptions for Longevity.* Laguna Beach, Calif.: Basic Health Publications, 2006.

Langer, Ellen J. *Counter Clockwise: Mindful Health and the Power of Possibility.* New York: Ballantine Books, 2009.

Langer, Ellen J. *Mindfulness*, 25th Anniversary Edition. Boston: Da Capo Lifelong Books, 2014.

Martins, Carla, Ph.D. *Mindfulness-Based Interventions for Older Adults: Evidence for Practice.* Philadelphia: Jessica Kingsley Publishers, 2014.

Parr, A.J. *Stop Negative Thinking in 7 Easy Steps (Understanding The Masters of Enlightenment: Eckhart Tolle, Dalai Lama, Krishnamurti and more!): 7 Lessons & 7 Exercises ... Beat Pessimism (The Secret of Now Book 6), Third Edition.* Madison, Wisc.: Grapevine Books (Ediciones De La Parra), 2016.

Santorelli, Saki. *Heal Thy Self: Lessons on Mindfulness in Medicine.* New York: Bell Tower, 1999.

Websites
For tips on learning how to meditate: http://meditation.org.au/online.asp

Endnotes
1. Ostir, Glenn V., Ph.D., Ivonne M. Berges, Ph.D., Kyriakos S. Markides, Ph.D. and Kenneth J. Ottenbacher, Ph.D. "Hypertension in Older Adults and the Role of Positive Emotions." *Psychosomatic Medicine.* 68:5 (Sep-Oct 2006), 727-733.
2. Klatz, Ronald, M.D. and Robert Goldman, M.D. "Healthy Aging: Natural Ways to Maintain a Youthful, Healthy Self." *To Your Health*: A MPA Media Publication. May 2009. http://www.toyourhealth.com/mpacms/tyh/article.php?id=1188
3. Phillip, John. "Targeted Nutrients Naturally Extend Telomere Length and Provide Anti-Aging Effect." *Natural News.* December 29, 2011. Accessed May 13, 2016.www.naturalnews.com/034513_telomeres_longevity_nutrition.html.
4. Shao, Bao-Mei, Wen Xu, Hui Dai, Pengfei Tu, Zhongjun Li and Xiao-Ming Gao. "A Study on the Immune Receptors for Polysaccharides from the Roots of Astragalus Membranaceus, A Chinese Medicinal Herb." *Biochemical and Biophysical Research Communication*: 320:4 (August 6, 2004). 1103-1111.
5. Phillip, John. "Targeted Nutrients Naturally Extend Telomere Length and Provide Anti-Aging Effect." Natural News. December 29, 2011. Accessed May 13, 2016. www.naturalnews.com/034513_telomeres_longevity_nutrition.html
6. Fenwick, Peter. "Scientific evidence for the efficacy of prayer." (2013). http://rcpsych.ac.uk/PDF/fenwick_%208_4_04.pdf
7. George, Simon, Ph.D. "Are We as Young as We Feel or as Old as We Think?" *Counseling Resource: Psychology, Philosophy and Real Life.* Accessed August 31, 2015.
8. Idem

Appendix

Muscle Testing Procedure

Clinical Kinesiology muscle testing is a simple and effective tool that can aid in your ability to understand the language of your body. You may wish to seek out a professional Clinical Kinesiologist in order to perform detailed muscle testing, but for more generalized and basic questions you can perform self-testing by following simple steps.

- Sit in a comfortable and sturdy chair.
- Remember to maintain a neutral state of mind.
- Perform an "indicator muscle test"* to determine your baseline strength by pushing on your dominant arm with your other hand. If you can easily resist moderate pressure, rest and then proceed.
- In order to test a food, supplement or similar item, you can place the item in your hand, lap or pocket and test for compatibility using the same format as the indicator muscle test.
  - If your body responds with a "strong" muscle test, you know that the food or supplement is compatible with your body.
  - If you find a "weak" muscle test in which your arm is easily pushed downward, you should avoid the food or other item.

> **Indicator Muscle Test***
> To perform an indicator muscle test, or test your arm's strength, hold one arm straightforward at shoulder height, parallel to the floor. Place the outstretched fingers on the other hand just slightly above the wrist of your testing arm. Keep the palm and fingers of the testing hand flat, just resting above the other wrist, not clutching it. Firmly hold the testing arm stationary as you then push down or toward the floor with the other (the pushing) hand. If you want to test yourself for compatibility with a food or supplement hold the item in your testing hand (the straight arm), or place it in your pocket. You should be able to discern between a weak and a strong muscle response. I strongly advise doing several practice tests to get the feel of the process.

Source: Levy, Susan L., D.C. *Your Body Can Talk, Second Edition.* Chino Valley, Ariz: Kalindi Press, 2014, 17.

Index

ACE inhibitors, 77
Acetyl L-carnitine, 92
Activated charcoal, 57, 118, 131-132
Acupuncture, 141, 147
Air filters, 110-111
Alcohol, 74, 78, 88, 148-149, 150, 168; also see Substance abuse
Alkaline, see pH
Allergies, 145
Alzheimer's Association, 164, 175
Alzheimer's disease, 39, 82, 129, 162-164, 166, 169
Amino acids, 58, 61, 64, 68-69, 82, 90, 92, 159, 161, 167, 172-173; also see L-Arginine, L-carnitine, L-carnosine and Protein
Anger, 27-28
Anona, 2
Antibodies, 92, 140
Antigens, 140, 142
Anti-inflammation, 98, 141, 149-152
Apple cider vinegar, 72, 117
Aqua Chi®, 119, 134
Asthma, 143-146
Astragalus, 131, 182
Autoimmune disease, 141, 145

B vitamins, 69, 72, 78, 82, 86, 88-89, 153, 158, 172, 182
Back pain, see Chronic back pain
Baking soda, 138
Bathing, 116-117
Beardall, Alan, xv-xvi, 147
Berkey®, 114, 134; also see Water filtration
Beta blockers, see ACE inhibitors
Beta-amyloid proteins, 164
Bile, 82
Biochemicals, 58

Blood clotting, 68, 77
Blood vessels, 63, 116, 165, 184
Bones, 68-69, 73, 84, 93
Brain, xv-xvi, 25, 39, 67, 89, 92, 95, 128-129
    and Inflammation, 145-146, 155
    and Longevity, 157-173
Bronchitis, 143
Buettner, Dan, 8

Caffeine, 75, 150, 167, 171
Calcium, 66-73, 75, 84
Calcium citrate, see Colloidal calcium
Cancer
    and Astragalus, 182
    Colon, 67, 126
    and Cruciferous vegetables, 82
    and GMOs, 70
    and Inflammation, 143
    and Mobility, 36
    Ovarian, 118
    and Toxins, 63, 118, 128
    and Trance minerals, 86
Carbohydrates, 57, 93-94
Carbon, 57-58
CedarCide®, 109, 134
Cell membrane, 73, 95, 173
Cerebral cortex, 160, 164
Cerebrum, 160
Charcoal, see Activated charcoal
Chemical elements, see Elements
Child, Julia, 14
Chiropractic, 46-48
Chloramine, 97, 105, 116
Chlorella pills, 130, 132
Chlorine, 84, 97, 117
Chlorophyll, 85
Chortega Indians, 1
Chronic back pain, 45

Cleansing clay, 130, 132
Clinical Kinesiology, xiv-xviii, 10, 176, 186-187; *also see* Muscle testing
   and Self-testing instructions, xvi-xix, 118, 193
   and Indicator muscle test, xviii, 194
   and New endeavors, 14-15
   and Trapped emotions, 26-28
   and Exercise, 48-49
   and Food, 59-60, 91, 112, 150
   and Supplement testing, 65, 71, 117, 123, 125-126, 153
   and Inflammation, 147-148
Cobalt, 84, 86-87, 158
Coconut oil, 96, 99, 121, 150-151, 154, 169
Coffee, 72, 75, 80, 100, 115, 150
Cognitive decline, 157-159
Cognitive impairment, 163-165
Colloidal calcium, 71
Colloidal silver, 117
Colon cancer, 67, 126
Colon cleansing, 126-127
Colon hydrotherapy, *see* Colonic
Colonic, 127; *also see* Colon cleansing
Concentrics, 42-43
Connective tissues, 58
Constipation, 89, 121, 125-126
Copper, 68, 84, 86, 158, 164
Coronary artery bypass graft, 177
Cosmetics, 63, 116, 128
C-reactive protein test, 147
Creutzfeldt-Jakob disease, 163
Cruciferous vegetables, 82-83; *also see* Sulforaphane
Cytokines, 139

Dairy products, 63, 69-70, 89, 171
Dementia, 145, 160, 163, 165, 168, 172-173
Deodorant, 116-118
Depression, 166-168
   and L-carnitine, 92
   and Calcium deficiency, 67
   and Cognitive decline, 157
   and Forgiveness, 29
   and Gratitude, 25
   and Grief, 27
   and Immobility, 36
   and Inflammation, 145

   and Leaky gut syndrome, 144
   and Tai chi, 39
   and Vitamin B_{12} deficiency, 89
   and Yoga, 42
Detoxification, 105-133, 164
   and Activated charcoal capsules, 57
   and Air, 109-111
   and Amino acids, 82
   and Bathing, 116-119
   and Colon cleansing, 121-127
   and Cosmetics, 127-128
   and Diet, 112-115, 150
   and Fasting, 114-115
   and Green tea, 182
   and Home environment, 108-109
   and Kidney, 131
   and L-carnosine, 92
   and Liver, 130
   and Lymphatic system, 131-132
   and Oil pulling, 121
   and Sleep, 128-129, 154
   and Vitamin B_{12}, 89
   and Whole body, 132
Diabetes, 169-170
   and Cognitive decline, 158
   and Inflammation, 141-143, 145
   and Minerals, 84
   and Mobility, 36
   and Potassium, 77, 80
   and Statin drugs, 166
   and Tai chi, 38
Diabetic ketoacidosis, 74, 79
Diet, 52-101, 159-161, 165, 183
Dietary minerals, *see* Nutrient minerals
Digestive blend recipe, 122-123
Digestive enzymes, 122-124, 153
DNA, 61, 74, 139, 149, 154, 180-181, 183
Dr. Bronner's liquid soap®, 109

Earthing, 38
Earthpaste®, 120
Egyptian Magic®, 128
Electrolyte replacement recipe, 79
Electrolytes, 76, 78-80, 84
Electromagnetic pollution, *see* Pollution
Elements, 53-55, 63-66, 85-87
Enemas, 126-127
Epsom salt, 81, 85, 117

Esmonde-White, Miranda, 42
Essentrics®, 42-43, 48
Exercise, 33-49, 80, 116; *also see* Essentrics®, Tai chi, Walking and Yoga

Fasting, 114-115
Fats, *see* Lipids and Phospholipids
Favao™, 102, 125, 134
Fecalith, 126
Fiber, 124-126
Fife, Bruce, 96, 121
Flexibility, 43, 46-48, 176, 178-179
Fluoride, 84, 97, 114, 120
Folic Acid, *see* B vitamins
Foot baths, *see* Hygiene
Forgiveness, 17, 27-29, 183, 185
Formaldehyde, 110-111, 128
Francina, Suza, 40

Gastrointestinal system, 39, 144, 184
Geronta, 2
Glimpse™, 128, 134
Glycerophosphorylcholine, 173
Glymphatic fluid, 162
Glymphatic system, 128, 162
GMOs, 70, 95, 100-101, 150
Gonzo Odor Eliminator™, 111, 134
Gout, 143
Grandma Moses, 13-14
Gratitude, 24-26, 29, 31, 176, 183, 185
Gravity deprivation syndrome, 34-35
Green tea, 151, 181-182
Grief, 27
Goldman, Robert, 179

Hair, 82, 86, 96, 128
Hair loss, 145
Hatha yoga, *see* Yoga
Head injury, 166
Heart, 66, 84, 92, 96, 144, 173
    and Calcium, 67-68
    and Coconut oil, 96
    and Disease, 36, 39, 72, 89, 126, 144, 165-166
    and Health, 29
    and Immobility, 35-36
    and L-carnitine, 92
    and Magnesium, 85

    and Potassium, 77-79
    and Selenium, 86
    and Tai chi, 39
    and Yoga, 41
HEPA filters, *see* Air filters
Herbal Dental Company®, 120, 134
Herbs, 154, 165
Humidifiers, 109-110
Huntington's disease, 163
Hwan-gap, 3
Hydrochloric acid 59, 72, 122
Hydrogen, 58-60
Hydroxyapatite, *see* Calcium phosphate
Hygiene, 116-122; *also see* Bathing, Colon cleansing, Deodorant, and Mouth care
    and Skin brush, 117
    and Apple cider vinegar, 117
    and Cosmetics, 127-128
    and Epsom salts, 117
    and Foot baths, 119
    and Magnesium flakes, 117
    and Sleep, 129
Hyperkalemia, 77-78

Ikigai, 7-10, 12, 24, 179
Ingalls Wilder, Laura, 13-14
Inflammation, 53, 137-138, 147-148, 162, 183
    and T-cells, 138-139
    Acute, 140-141
    Brain, 145-146
    Chronic, 138, 140-141, 143
    and Clinical Kinesiology, 147-148
    and C-reactive protein test, 148
    and Digestive enzymes, 153
    and Foods, 150-151
    and Herbs, 154
    and Leaky gut syndrome, 142-145
    and Nutritional supplements, 153
    and Omega 6, 96
    Reduction, 148-155
    and Sleep, 155
    Toxic, 140-141
    and Triggers, 141-142
    Whole body, 143
    and Xanthones, 151-152
International Association for Colon Hydrotherapy, 127
Iodine, 86

Iron, 86

Jerusalem artichokes, 170
Juice fasting, *see* Fasting
Juni™, 128, 134

Kidneys, 68, 74, 77-80, 131
Klatz, Ronald, 179
KohCui, 3
Kübler-Ross, Elizabeth, 27

Language, 30, 42, 173-174, 176
L-Arginine, 63
L-carnitine, 92, 182
L-carnosine, 92
Leaky gut syndrome, 142-145, 153
Levine, James A., 36, 43
Lily Organics®, 128
Lipids, 73, 95-96 *also see* Phospholipids
Liver, 184; *also see* Liver flush
   and Alcohol, 168
   and Amino acids, 82
   and Detox, 130
   and Leaky gut syndrome, 144
   and Lemon juice, 114
   and Sleep, 128
   and Toxins, 116
Liver flush, 130
Longevity, 10; *also see* Youthing
   and Amino acids, 92
   and Brain, 157-173
   and Detox, 105-133
   and DNA, 181, 183
   and Hydrogen, 60
   and Inflammation, 142
   and Nicoyan people, 2
   and Nutrients, 96
   and Okinawans, 8
   and Sense of purpose, 2, 7
   and Sleep, 149, 154
   and Spirituality, 185-186
   and Telomeres, 180, 183
Lotion, 116, 120, 128; *also see* Juni™
Lungs, 35, 42, 109, 147
Lupus, 141-142, 145
Lymphatic massage, 131
Lymphatic system, 39, 131, 162

Macronutrients, 53, 56, 90-91; *also see* Carbohydrates, Lipids, and Protein
Magnesium, 85
Manganese, 86
Mangosteen, 151-152
Marañón, 2
Medication, 141-142, 146, 162; *also see* ACE inhibitors and Statins
   Calcium, 72-73
   and Dementia, 163
   and Foot baths, 119
   and Grapefruit juice, 60
   Phosphorus, 76
   Potassium, 77, 80
   and Tap water, 107
Meditation, 37, 172, 178-179, 186-189; *also see* Tai chi and Youthing: A Meditation
Memory, 39, 92, 108, 144, 157, 160-164, 172-174, 184-185
Metabolism, 44, 64, 77, 87, 90, 133
Methylcobalamin, *see* Vitamins
Micronutrients, 53, 64-89, 114; *also see* Nutrient minerals and Vitamins
Mild traumatic brain injury (MTBI), 157, 174
Milk, 69-70, 99, 102-103
Mind-body connection, 15, 190
Mindfulness, 177-178, 183, 186
Minerals, *see* Nutrient minerals
Mitochondria, 73, 80
Mobility, 24, 41, 46, 177, 188
Molybdenum, 84
Mood disorders, 166-168
Morse, Robert S., 115
MoSo Bags®, 11
Mouth care, 120-121
Movement, *see* Exercise
Multipure®, 114, 134; *also see* Water filtration
Muscle degeneration, 77
Muscle Testing, xv-xvii, 5, 49, 71, 118, 188, 193
Myopathies, 143; *also see* Neuropathy

NEAT (non-exercise activity thermogenesis), 36
Neurofibrillary tangles, 164
Neurons, 160-161, 172
Neuropathy, 88, 143

Niacin, *see* B vitamins
Nitrogen, 61-63
Nitrogen rich fertilizer recipe, 62
Non-REM sleep, 162
Nutrients, *see* Macronutrients and Micronutrients
Nuts and seeds, 70, 74, 91, 98, 183

Oil pulling, 121
Okinawans, 3, 7-8, 97
Omega 3, 149, 153
Omega 6, 96
Organic fabrics, 108-109
Organic Triple Fiber, 125
Oxygen, 55-56; *also see* Air filters and Oxygen deficiency
   and Air, 109-112
   and Blood, 86, 184
   and Brain, 160
   and Deficiency, 56, 160
   and Plants, 110-112
   and Potassium, 77
   and Trace minerals, 86

Parkinson's disease, 39, 42, 45, 80, 82-83
Parsons Burkitt, Denis, 124-125
Patients and Stories
   Allorah Jo, 13
   Alyssa Mae, 19-21
   Consuela, 107-108, 152-153
   Guillermo and Benita, 1-2
   Maria and Walter, 22-23
   Ruth, 146-147
pH, 59-60, 74, 76, 114, 117, 122
Phosphatidyl serine, 173
Phospholipids, 73, 173
Phosphorus, 73-76
PiperWai, 118, 134
Pollution, 38, 107, 111, 142, 171
Potassium, 67, 76-80
Pranayama, 40, 55
Primal Pit Paste™, 118, 135
Processed foods, 94-95, 112, 125, 149, 172
Protein powder, 91-92; *also see* Favo™
Protein 90-93; *also see* Amino Acids, Beta-amyloid proteins, C-reactive protein test, and Tau proteins
   and Cytokines, 139
   and Alzheimer's disease, 129, 162, 164
   and Blood sugar, 90
   and Digestive enzymes, 59
   and Microwave oven, 113
   and Red blood cells, 56
   and Water, 1
Pyridoxine, *see* B vitamins

Qi Gong, *see* Tai chi
Quercetin, 153

Recombinant bovine growth hormone (rbGH), 70
Recombinant bovine somatotrropin (rBST), 70
Rhabdomyolysis, 77
Rheumatoid arthritis, 141, 145
RNA, 61, 74
Ryukyuan, 3

Salt, *see* Sodium
Semisupercentenarians, 1
Serine, 82, 173
Shampoo, 111, 128, 134; *also see* Juni™
Simple tooth powder recipe, 120
Skin, 116, 128, 184; *also see* Lotion
   and Calcium, 69
   and Carbon, 58
   and Cleanser, 114, 120, 128
   and Copper, 84, 86
   and Exfoliant, 119
   and Fats, 95
   and Fatty acids, 96
   and L-carosine, 92
   and Leaky gut syndrome, 145
   and Multi-minerals, 67
   and Potassium, 78
   and Protein, 93
   and Skin brushing, 117, 132
   and Sleep, 149, 154
   and Smoking, 87
   and Sulfur, 81-82
   and Tai chi, 38
   and Toxins, 109
   and Vitamin C, 87
   and Water, 97
Sleep, 10, 33, 96-97, 162
   and Calcium, 67

Sleep (*continued*)
   and Deficiency, 171-172
   and Detox, 128-129
   and Gratitude, 25
   and Inflammation, 149, 154
   and Tai chi, 38
   and Telomeres, 183
   and Vitamin B_{12}, 89
Small intestine, 142
Soap, 109, 134; *also see* Skin care and Dr. Bronner's liquid soap
Sodium, 76, 78, 80
Sodium fluoride, 84, 97, 100, 120
Spinal cord, 82, 160, 162-163
Spinal fluid, 162
Spirulina pills, 131
Statins, 77, 157, 165-166
Stereotypes, 18, 30-31
Stroke, 77-78, 157, 165, 173, 177
Substance abuse, 25, 167-168
Sulforaphane, 82-83
Sulfur, 81-83, 154, 181

Tai chi, 37-39, 48
Talcum powder, 118
Tap water, 97, 105, 107, 116
Tau proteins, 164
T-cells, 139
Teeth, 57, 68, 72-73, 88, 120-121, 145; *also see* Mouth Care
Telomerase, 182
Telomeres, 92, 180-183,
Therapeutic ultrasound, 141
Thiamine, *see* B vitamins
Thymus gland, 86, 138
Tobacco, 73, 143, 149, 165, 167, 183
Toothpaste 120, 134; *also see* Earthpaste®, Mouth care and Simple tooth powder recipe
Toxins, 106-107, 133, 142, 162
   and Activated charcoal tablets, 57
   and Alzheimer's disease, 129
   and Amino acids, 82

and Diet, 10, 112-113
and Environment, 108-111, 159
and Hygiene products, 116-122
and Muscle response, xvii
and Sleep, 128-129
and Water, 113-114, 149
Trace elements, 85-86
Trichloroethylene, 111
Tryptophan, 92, 171, 182
Turmeric, 83, 154, 165, 181

Ultrasound, *see* Therapeutic ultrasound

Vernikos, Joan, 33-35, 43
Vitamins 53, 57-58, 64, 82, 87-89, 95, 149, 172; *also see* B vitamins
   Vitamin A, 72, 88
   Vitamin C, 2, 68, 72, 87-88, 116-117, 150, 158, 182
   Vitamin D, 68, 75, 78, 158, 167
   Vitamin E, 86, 158, 182
   Vitamin K, 68-69

Walking, 33-36, 43-46, 55, 178
Water, 96-100, 105-107, 112-119, 149, 170; *also see* Bathing and Water filtration
Water filtration, 114-117; *also see* Multipure® and Berkey®
Wellness Mama, 128, 134
White blood cells, 138-140

Xango juice, 103, 152-153, 156
Xanthones, 151-152

Yahrzeit, 4-5
Yoga, 40-41, 49
Youthing, 1, 3-4, 88, 176-190; *also see* Youthing: A Meditation
Youthing: A Meditation, 188-190

Zakein, 4
ZEROREZ®, 109, 135
Zinc, 68, 72, 78, 84, 86, 158, 182

Previous Book by Doctor Susan L. Levy

Your Body Can Talk, 2nd Edition
ISBN: 978-1-935826-36-1

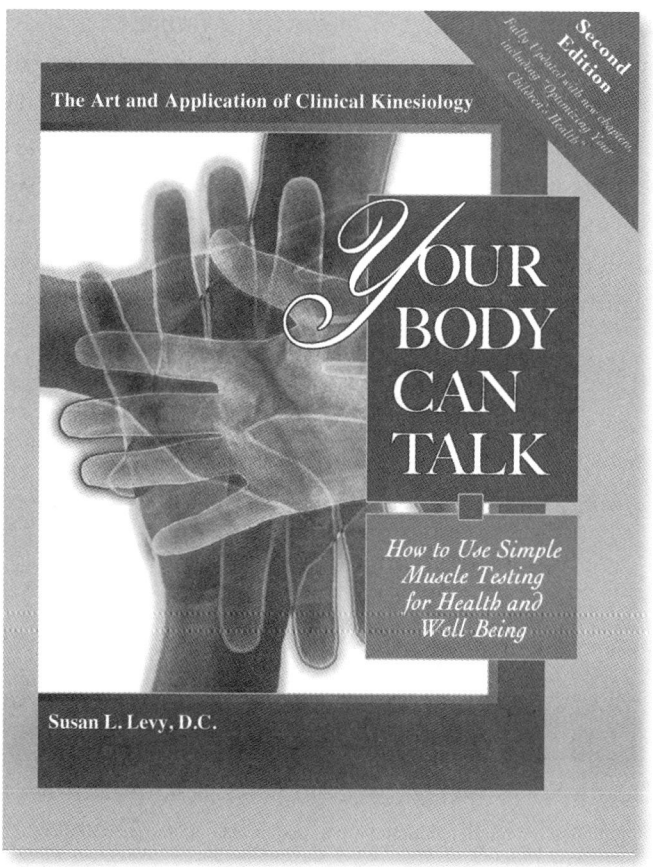

To connect with Dr. Levy online:
WEBSITE: http://www.yourbodycantalk.com/
FACEBOOK: https://www.facebook.com/YourBodyCanTalk/

About the Author

Susan L. Levy, D.C. has extensive training in massage, polarity therapy, nutrition, herbology, is a registered nurse, a Chiropractor, and is certified in acupuncture by the International Academy of Medical Acupuncture. Dr. Levy's positive, gentle, healing presence promotes an alternative method for restoring and maintaining your health. She approaches the broad topics of human body function and dysfunction from several vantage points, including multiple health care disciplines, traditions, and philosophies. Her popular seminars, newsletters and articles emphasize natural health care through balance, harmony, expertise and love. She continues to research pathways to assist her patients as expediently as possible, and is eager to share this remarkable approach with her colleagues. She lives in Colorado where she was named Chiropractor of the Year in 1985.

CONTACT
http://www.yourbodycantalk.com/
https://www.facebook.com/YourBodyCanTalk/
Phone: 1-800-770-6704

About Kalindi Press

Kalindi Press, an affiliate of **Hohm Press**, proudly offers books in natural health and nutrition, as well as the acclaimed Family and World Health Series for children and parents, covering such themes as nutrition, dental health, reading, and environmental education.

CONTACT AND TO ORDER
Kalindi Press / Hohm Press, PO Box 4410, Chino Valley, Arizona, 86323, USA.
800-381-2700 / 928-636-3331
publisher@hohmpress.com
www.kalindipress.com